ALONE TOGETHER

Be With The People You Love, Even If You Can't Set Foot In The Hospital

Written By

JANET GREENWALD
&
LAURA GREENWALD

Published by Get Your Stuff Together
Lion and The Rock Entertainment

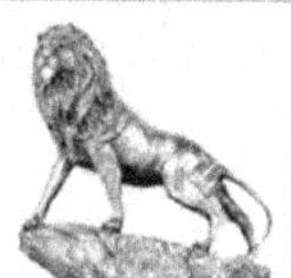

For information about special discounts and bulk purchases go to www.getyourstufftogether.com
or email us at corpsales@getyourstufftogether.com

Manufactured in the United States of America

ISBN: 979-8665798172

Table Of Contents

FOREWORD

In 2005, when I created the ICE, In Case of Emergency concept and campaign little did I know ICE would become a global phenomenon and still running just as strong more than a decade later.

Little did I realise then also was that my incredibly simple idea would take me on travels far and wide, meeting other like-minded individuals who also shared my aspirations.

When Laura and Janet Greenwald entered my life, it quickly became evident this entrepreneurial team were not satisfied with merely helping others prepare for the unexpected; they were and are passionate about a much wider holistic approach. After all, if we can make the unexpected any less unpleasant or devastating for ourselves and our loved ones, why stop there?

In providing a comprehensive portfolio of emergency preparedness material for all, Laura and Janet are empowering each of us; whichever method we choose to utilise for making a difference to outcomes we just cannot see coming.

As a paramedic, my shifts were littered with those I attended and who were conscious stating *"I didn't think I'd be in this position today when I woke."*

Remember, none of us 'likes' to be harbingers of doom but the reality is in considering a plan, we can more easily forget about the possibilities, safe in the knowledge we are in at least some way, prepared.

Bob Brotchie
Award Winning Founder of ICE, Former UK Paramedic
www.incaseofemergency.org

Before You Begin

Go to http://getyourstufftogether.com/gystcovid/gystcoviddownloads.zip to download all of the tools, documents and forms that come along with this book. You can either print them out and fill them in by hand, or open them and fill them out on your computer before saving and printing the completed form. Whatever is easier for you.

Be sure to save the downloads to your computer desktop so that you can quickly grab them and use them as we work through the book.

Depending on your computer, the materials may be in a ZIP file. Here's how to use it.

How To Download a ZIP file
To download a zip file, right click on the link, choose "Save Target As", and save the Zip file to your desktop.

How To Open a ZIP File
A ZIP file is a folder that holds all of your documents zipped up inside for easy downloading. Once you download it, you'll see a little icon that looks like a file box. Double clicking on it, it will open and all the files will appear.

You can extract the documents one of two ways: 1) Click the extract button and all of the files will be extracted from the box and land on your desktop. 2) Highlight all the files, click CTRL +C to copy them and then CTRL+V to paste them onto your desktop.

How to Get a Copy of Adobe's Free Adobe Reader PDF Software
Go to www.adobe.com and follow the instructions to download the latest free PDF software from their website.

Introduction

People are always asking us what they can do to keep the people they love safe while they're in the hospital.

Usually our advice is pretty straightforward. Go to the hospital with them and don't leave them alone. Just pitch a tent at their bedside and get comfortable.

Okay, there's a little more to it than that. But THAT was before Coronavirus reared its ugly head.

Now every hospital here in the U.S. and around the world has a new mandate to keep everyone as safe as possible.

No visitors. No family. No argument.

Now what?

What can you do to keep someone you love as safe and connected as possible if they end up in the hospital in the middle of the pandemic?

A lot more than you think.

The good news is that with the tools and tips in this book, along with a little prep work, you can keep your loved one and her medical staff safety at arm's length while keeping a pulse on her and her condition.

Whether that person has COVID-19 or is hospitalized for some other reason, like surgery, childbirth or having treatment for chronic conditions, the key is making it easy for the hospital to stay connected with you and your family.

Quick Start

Hospital staffs are overworked and overburdened. The last thing they're going to do right now is to remember to call a patient's family to give them an update or let them talk to the patient ESPECIALLY if they have to figure out who to call or go looking for your number.

The other thing they won't have time to do is search for a list of your loved one's past medical conditions or current medications, if they're not already in their system. They're going to concentrate on treating their current condition. Which is fine until something goes wrong.

That's why it's so important for you to make it EASY for them using the instructions and tools in this book.

How? With these three things:

A Medical History Form
And ICE Contact
A page called Information Central, to pull it all together.

So let's get started.

Your family probably fits into one of three categories:

Critical:
You have family members in the hospital or in immediate danger of being hospitalized. You need the quickest way possible to keep yourself connected with your loved ones and their medical staff.

Vital:
Your family members have been exposed to the virus and are under quarantine, but aren't symptomatic. You have a few days to put together everything your loved ones would need if they had to be hospitalized.

Just Want To Be Prepared:
You want to use the downtime you have while sheltering at home, to put together the information you would need for every member of your household, just in case.

Here's What You Need To Do

Critical

1. Choose a **Point Person** for your family (page 6).

2. Fill out the **Medical History Form** (page 15) for members of your family who are ill.

3. Make a **2 Minute ICE Contact** (page 9) for each of those family members.

4. Read the section on **Different Ways You Can Communicate With Your Family Member** (page 21).

5. Then fill in an **Information Central** page (page 18) for each one of them.

Once you've completed these steps, print or make two copies of the Medical History Forms and Information Central pages. Keep one at home and place one set in an envelope to send with your loved one to the hospital. **Tuck in a note asking the nursing staff to tape the Information Central page to the head of your loved one's bed.**

Remember that you might not be able to accompany them into the hospital, so write on the envelope in large letters: **Attention nursing staff for "PATIENT'S NAME". Important information enclosed. Please open and read. Thank you!**

If your loved one is already hospitalized, call his/her nurse and tell them that you want to send over important information about the patient and ask if you can email it over to them. If they balk, tell them it includes vital information about their medical history and special communication needs.   Make sure that your loved one's smartphone or tablet and cord/charger, accompany them to the hospital. That phone might be the only way that you'll be able to communicate with your loved one while they're at the hospital. In fact, if you have a portable power charger, send that along as well.

It might not be a bad idea to put your loved one's name on the phone, cord and charger, just to be safe.

Once you're finished, go ahead and complete the steps below for yourself and the other members of your family.

Vital

Complete the steps above for each member of your family who is in danger of contracting the virus. Then…

Create a **Smart Contact** (page 38) on your own phone for each of those family members.

We've also included a form so everyone in your home can list his or her **Social Media and Web Passwords** (page 41), in case you need to use them, when your loved one is unable to communicate.

Just Want To Be Prepared

Complete the steps above for each member of your family. Then…

Since you have time, make a full **ICE Contact** (page 24) for each member of the family instead of the 2 minute version.

Read the section on **Making Your Family Findable** (page 42)

Point Person

An overworked hospital staff will be much more likely to talk to and keep in touch, with one, calm, easy to talk to person, rather than ten people demanding information ten times a day.

Since you're the person reading this book, the point person for your family is probably you. Or if you've been exposed to the virus and are being proactive, you'll probably want to make your spouse, parent or adult child your point person. In any case, we suggest choosing one main person who will stay in contact with the hospital, the patient and the rest of the family.

The Point Person's name goes in the first position of the Information Central page. His or her contact information should also be the main ICE Contact on the patient's phone. Easy to find, easy to call.

Now one caveat. COVID-19 has been striking entire families, sending different members to the hospital, sometimes unexpectedly. During the pandemic, it might be wise to name alternate point people on your family's Information Central pages, just in case the main person ends up falling ill.

Another smart idea is to name a relative or close friend who lives outside of your immediate area as your alternate Point Person. Not only are they just as able to stay in touch via phone and internet, but if they're not in an area that's been hard hit, they're less likely to end up in the hospital themselves.

The last few months have been such a crazy time for the world. For us, one of the things that keeps us centered the most is praying Psalm 91, the Psalm of protection, over ourselves, our family and our friends.

It's All About Communication

This is one of the most important and most personal books that we've ever written. Why? Because we found out the hard way, how vital it is to have this part of our lives absolutely organized, armor-plated, undefeatable and secure.

I'll never forget the day I realized it wasn't.

My grandmother Elaine Sullivan was an active seventy-one year old living on her own in Chicago. One day while getting ready to take a bath, she slipped and fell, striking her head and mouth on the side of the tub. Her neighbors realized they hadn't seen her all day and called the paramedics, who went in and found her, conscious, but unable to speak.

She was taken to a hospital where she had previously been a patient, she had Medicare, supplemental insurance and everything she needed. Or so we thought.

Even though she was stable, injuries to her mouth made her unable to speak for herself. Over the next few days, after a series of serious medical errors and a critical drug interaction, her condition worsened.

My mom Janet and I had no idea what was happening. We were working back in Los Angeles, and since Grandma was scheduled to leave on vacation that day, we weren't expecting to hear from her. Despite the fact that the hospital had our contact information, they waited until she slipped into critical condition, six and a half days later, to call us. By the time they did, it was too late. We weren't able to get to her before she passed away, unnecessarily and alone.

As we began to put the pieces together to find out what actually happened, we realized that there were no laws regulating next of kin notification. So we swooped in and led the charge to create and enact three Next of Kin laws in Illinois and California.

What we *didn't* realize, is that having a law doesn't necessarily mean that every hospital will suddenly start taking the time to call a patient's family, especially if that information isn't right at their fingertips. Maybe we would have realized that, if we'd taken a breath and though about it. But instead, we just jumped in with both feet ready to change the world.

We did to a point – the law and our Notify In 7 Training System have definitely saved lives. But to this day, we still get letters from families telling us that their dad or son or daughter died alone because a hospital neglected to find and call their next of kin.

And that's when it dawned on us. A better solution.

Grandma died because the hospital gave her medication that caused a fatal interaction with a prescription she was already taking. Why? Because the doctors treating her didn't have her medical or prescription drug history at their fingertips.

Which means that there is one simple thing that would have prevented her death.

An ICE Contact.

An in case of emergency contact that you place on your smartphone detailing your emergency contacts along with basic medical, prescription drug and allergy information.

Since then, through our book *Connected*, our blog and our revolutionary Smart Contact and 2 Minute ICE Contact, we've become the foremost ICE educators in America. More than 1.3 million families have used our books and materials to keep themselves and the people they love safe and sound.

The moral of the story? You never know what piece of information, no matter how small, might save the life of someone you love. Taking a few minutes to tuck your information into the contacts of your smartphone is the perfect first step.

The Two Minute ICE Contact | iPhone

ICE contacts are kind of our thing. You see my grandma Elaine passed away because a Chicago hospital neglected to call and tell Mom and I that she had fallen at home and was unable to communicate because she hit her mouth. By the time they called us, she had slipped into critical condition. The nurses refused to get a phone to her so that we could talk to her one last time and before we could even get on the plane, she passed away, alone.

The reason? The hospital gave her a drug that interacted with when she was already taking. Not only could we have told them she had been on that medication, but a simple ICE Contact with the name of that drug would have saved her life.

Although ICE Contacts usually belong on your smartphone, during the Coronavirus outbreak, it's just as important to have that information readily available on a piece of paper that hospital personnel can see posted on your loved one's headboard.

CoVID-19 patients, might be admitted to a hospital with doctors who don't know them, or who don't have their medical records.

So once you're finished completing a Two Minute ICE Contact for them, make sure you jot down the names and information for their main contacts (including you) on the Information Central page along with their basic medical history in the medical history form, to send along with them to the hospital.

The Two Minute ICE Contact that follows is a basic contact that will do nicely, until you have the time to do a detailed one. You'll find instructions for a full contact for your particular phone later in the book.

What Is A Two Minute ICE Contact?

During Hurricane Katrina, so many people were injured & separated from their families, that emergency workers came up with the idea of putting an ICE – In Case Of Emergency – contact in their cell phones. Now, hospitals worldwide, check patient's phones for their ICE contact, to locate their next of kin.

Problem is, an ICE Contact can take five or ten minutes to put into your iPhone. Not a lot of time, but when you're in between tasks and want to get it done while you're thinking about it – something we definitely suggest – five or ten minutes can be longer than you really have time for.

Not to worry. That's why we created the two minute version. Everything thing you absolutely need to have in your contact, until you have a few extra minutes to turn your quickie ICE Contact into a real lfesaver.

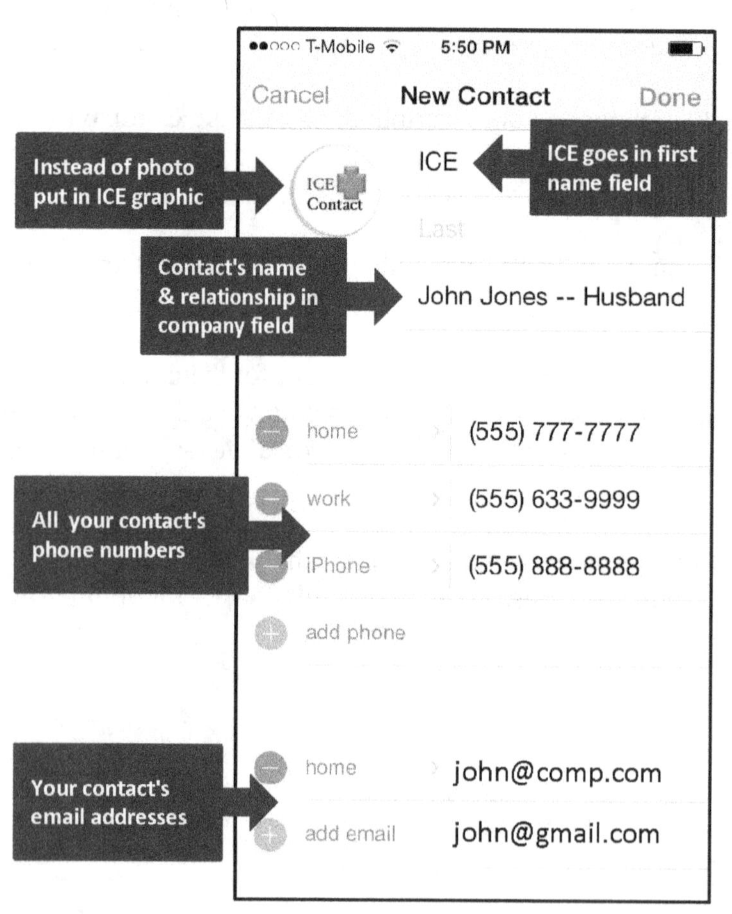

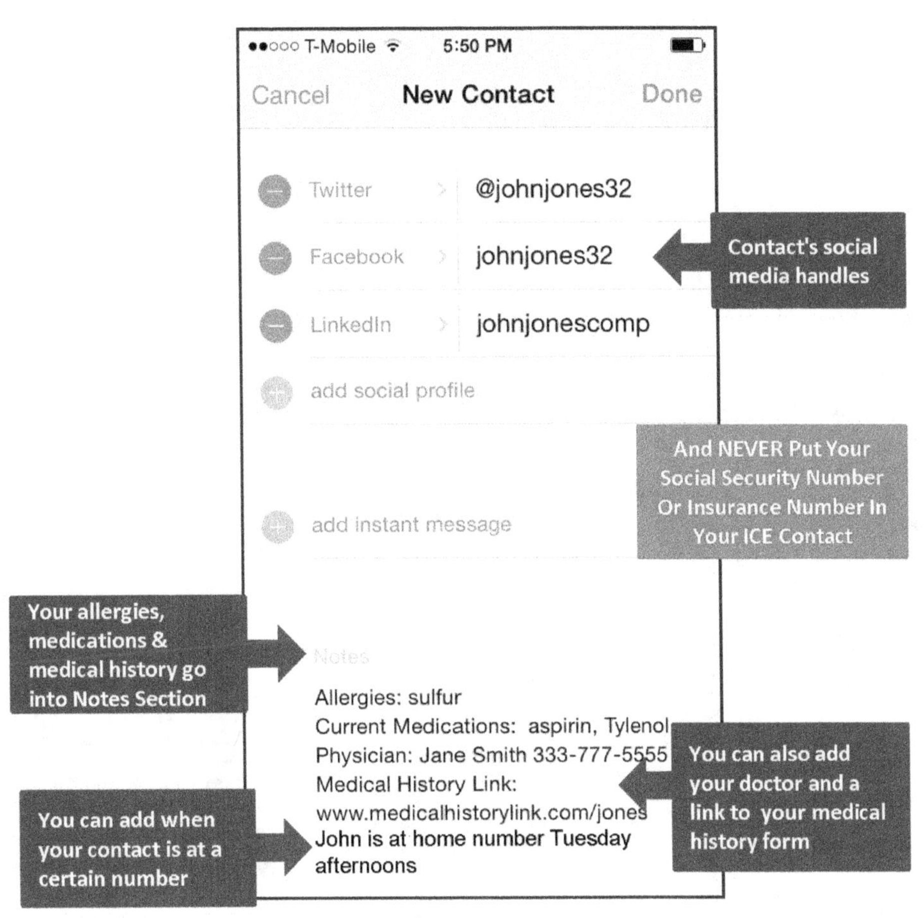

●●○○○ T-Mobile   5:50 PM
Cancel   New Contact   Done
Twitter   @johnjones32
Facebook   johnjones32
LinkedIn   johnjonescomp
add social profile
add instant message
Notes
Allergies: sulfur
Current Medications: aspirin, Tylenol
Physician: Jane Smith 333-777-5555
Medical History Link:
www.medicalhistorylink.com/jones
John is at home number Tuesday
afternoons
Contact's social media handles
And NEVER Put Your Social Security Number Or Insurance Number In Your ICE Contact
Your allergies, medications & medical history go into Notes Section
You can also add your doctor and a link to your medical history form
You can add when your contact is at a certain number

The Two Minute ICE Contact | Samsung Galaxy

GET YOUR STUFF TOGETHER

What Is A Two Minute ICE Contact?

During Hurricane Katrina, so many people were injured & separated from their families, that emergency workers came up with the idea of putting an ICE – In Case Of Emergency – contact in their cell phones. Now, hospitals worldwide, check patient's phones for their ICE contact, to locate their next of kin.

Problem is, an ICE Contact can take five or ten minutes to put into your iPhone. Not a lot of time, but when you're in between tasks and want to get it done while you're thinking about it – something we definitely suggest – five or ten minutes can be longer than you really have time for.

Not to worry. That's why we created the two minute version. Everything thing you absolutely need to have in your contact, until you have a few extra minutes to turn your quickie ICE Contact into a real lfesaver.

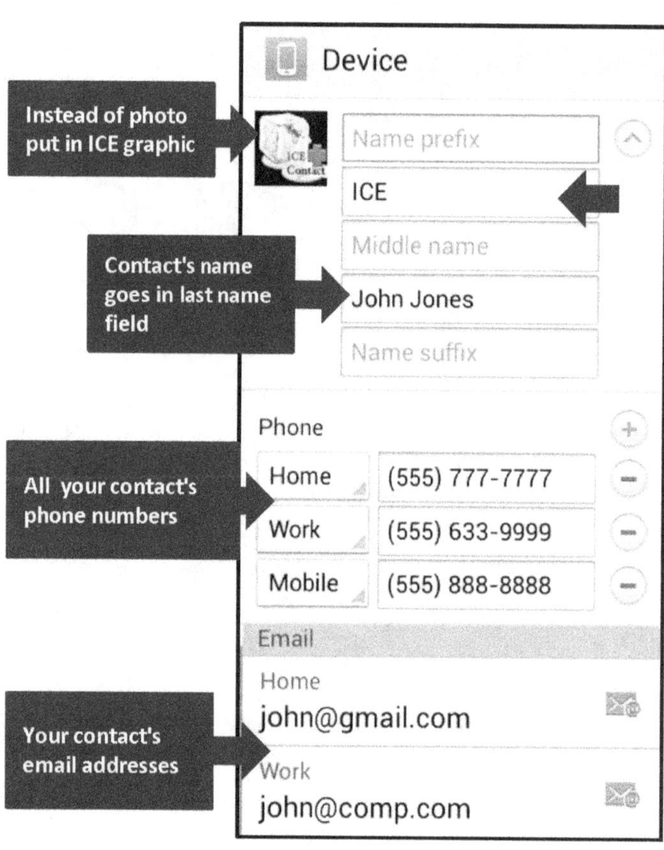

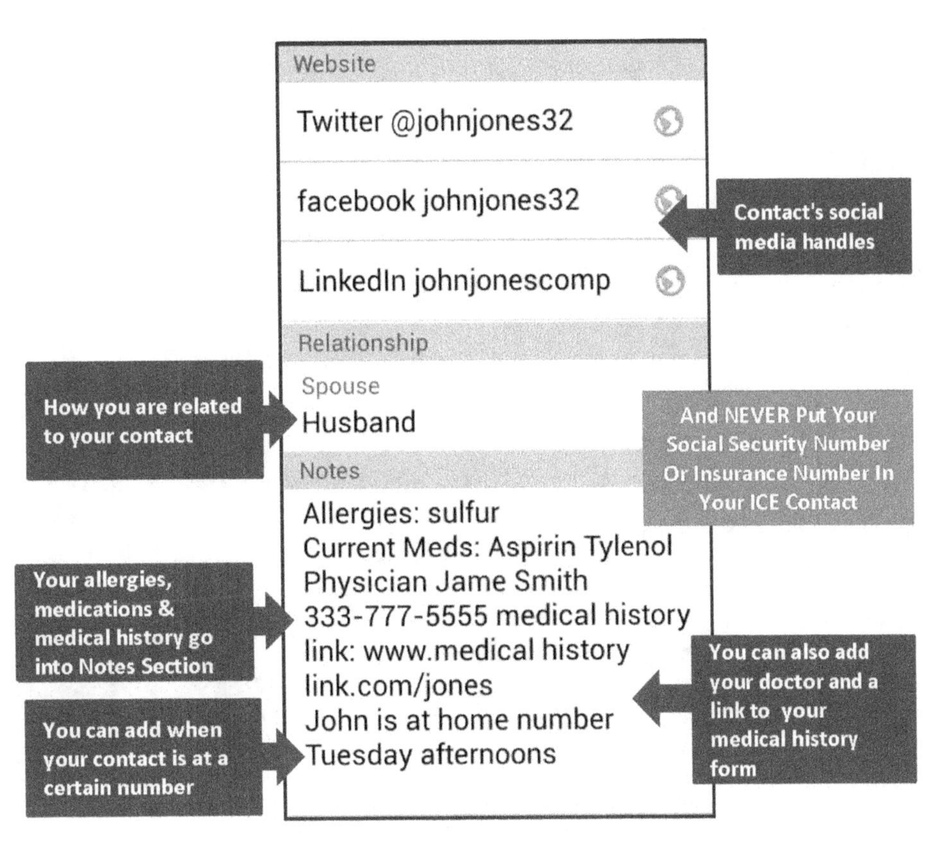
Website
Twitter @johnjones32
facebook johnjones32
LinkedIn johnjonescomp
Relationship
Spouse
Husband
Notes
Allergies: sulfur
Current Meds: Aspirin Tylenol
Physician Jame Smith
333-777-5555 medical history
link: www.medical history
link.com/jones
John is at home number
Tuesday afternoons
Contact's social media handles
How you are related to your contact
And NEVER Put Your Social Security Number Or Insurance Number In Your ICE Contact
Your allergies, medications & medical history go into Notes Section
You can also add your doctor and a link to your medical history form
You can add when your contact is at a certain number

How To Keep Your Medical Information At Your Fingertips

The Medical History Form gives you a place to record your family member's medical history, allergies, the medications they're taking, vitamins and their insurance information along with the names of their physicians and healthcare providers.

In an emergency, especially in the middle of the pandemic, a person in need of life-saving treatment can end up in any hospital – not necessarily the one with the personal physician and medical records.

This medical history form will give your loved one's medical staff all of the information they need to treat the people you love with their specific medical history in mind.

You'll find a version of this form in the back of this book and an editable version of the form in the downloadable files. Go ahead and open it or print it and fill it out on the computer or by hand. Once you're finished, put it to the side until you're ready to gather the documents you need to send to the hospital with the person you love.

Your Mission, Should You Choose To Accept It...

...is to set up a Medical Information Form for each member of your family. Open the Medical Information Forms (you'll find them inside the Backup Plan Forms you downloaded at the beginning of the book) and let's get started.

What Info Am I Going To Need?   1

Grab a pencil and paper and jot down the types of medical information you have for each member of the family.

This includes your family's medical history, medical information, names of everyone's physicians, specialists, dentists, optometrists and other health care providers and current and past prescriptions.

What Would You Need A Doctor To Know?   2

Close your eyes for a moment & imagine that you're sitting in the ER with everyone in your house. One by one, imagine that your spouse and other family members has an injury, like a broken arm, or needs emergency surgery. The doctor – who doesn't know you or your family's unique medical needs – walks through the door.

What does this doctor need to know about them? Jot down all of the things that just went through your mind. Old injuries, allergies, surgeries, anything you think is important.

Locate & Gather All The Information You Have   3

Using those notes and the list you completed in Step 1, **locate** and **gather** all of the medical information you have at home, along with your address book or contact information for physicians and the people you'll be using for emergency contacts.

Create Your Family's Medical History Forms   4

Grab the Medical Information Form you downloaded earlier and create one for each adult and child in your family, adding all of the information you've located.

Choosing Your Emergency Contacts 5

Choose and name at least 3 emergency contacts for each person, including yourself.
- Main Emergency Contact: If you are married, include your spouse on your form and yourself on your spouse's form. For your children, this would be you and your spouse.
- 2nd Contact: should be a nearby relative or good friend who you would trust enough to make informed choices on your behalf, if necessary.
- 3rd Contact: should be an out of town/out of state relative or friend.

Anything Else To Add? 6

Is there any other information you need, to deal with a medical emergency while evacuated or away from home? If so, scan or make copies of that information and place it in the same folder as your completed medical history forms.

And while you're at it, don't forget to put ICE (In Case Of Emergency) Contacts in your and your family's smartphones along with a copy or link to your medical history forms. That way if you ever need quick access to a family member's medical history you'll have it right at your fingertips. Need instructions on ICE Contacts? Just go to that section of the book.

Now For Safekeeping... 7

Print, scan or make three copies of the form you just completed, along with the documents or other materials you need to have grabbable, and store them in at least **three** secure, damage-proof locations. That way if one or two of the locations are inaccessible, you'll still be able to grab the information you need.

You should also consider attaching the forms to your emergency contact cards (school & work) as well as placing a set on a secure web server and putting a link to them in your smartphone, so you'll always have your medical history forms at your fingertips wherever you are.

Information Central

Information Central gives doctors, nurses and the hospital staff the information they need to keep you connected to the person you love. It also gives them a right-on-the-bed summary of their medical history, contacts and the way you and they prefer to communicate, for example FaceTime versus a phone call.

All you have to do is ask the medical team tape it to the head of your loved one's bed so they can refer to it and use it often.

Since you probably won't be able to be there when the person you love is admitted, the first time you talk to the medical staff, make sure that you ask them to open the envelope that accompanied them to the hospital, tape the Information Central page to the head of their bed and add the information on their Medical History Form to their chart.

Just print the Information Central page from the book or from the downloads and fill it out. You'll find a sample of a completed version, on the next page.

Hi, My Name Is:

My Next Of Kin Contacts

Point Person For Family:

Alternate Contact One:

Alternate Contact Two:

My Communications Preferences

I would like to talk to ________ twice a day, via

If I'm not able to communicate myself, please update __________ twice a day on my condition. If things become critical please contact ________ immediately and hold the phone to my ear so that ____________ can speak to me.

Allergies, Prescription Drugs, Pre-Existing Conditions and Other Vital Medical History

Allergies   Prescriptions I am Currently Taking:

Birthmarks & Other Distinguishing Marks & Scars:

Pre-Existing Conditions: Primary Care/Main Physicians:

All other information can be found in my Medical History Form.

Hi, My Name Is: Parker Smith

My Next Of Kin Contacts	My Communications Preferences
Point Person For Family: Jane Smith (wife) cell 444-675-9989 home 888-000-7777 jane@smith.com Skype @janesmith Facebook @janesmithfb **Alternate Contact One:** Jim Smith (son) cell 444-866-7777 home 888-555-1212 jimsmith@bac.com Skype @bacjim Facebook @jimsconcrete **Alternate Contact Two:** Jim Smith (son) cell 444-866-7777 home 888-555-1212 jimsmith@bac.com Skype @bacjim Facebook @jimsconcrete	I would like to talk to Jane twice a day, on Skype or if that's not possible, on the phone. If I'm not able to communicate myself, please update Jane twice a day on my condition. If things become **critical** please contact Jane **immediately** and hold the phone to my ear so that **Jane & my family can speak to me.**

Allergies, Prescription Drugs, Pre-Existing Conditions and Other Vital Medical History

Allergies: Sulfur, Penicillin   Prescriptions I am Currently Taking: Calan, Vitamin C, Sudafed

Birthmarks & Other Distinguishing Marks & Scars: Birthmark upper right leg, appendix scar

Pre-Existing Conditions: Flat Feet   Primary Care/Main Physicians: Dr. Patricia Reese 555-333-7878

All other information can be found in my Medical History Form.

Different Ways To Communicate With The Person You Love

On the phone

This is probably the easiest way to talk to a loved one in the hospital. Even if he or she can't speak, a member of the medical staff can always put the phone up to their ear or put the call on speaker so you can talk to them.

I don't have to tell you what a difference hearing a familiar voice on the phone can make for someone who is unconscious or unresponsive. After my Grandma's stroke, the moment she heard Mom's and my voices on the phone, her eyes snapped open and she came out of her coma. Enough said.

FaceTime/Skype/Webex/Zoom

Video calls are a great way to stay in touch with anyone in the hospital. One of the worst things about not being able to be at someone's bedside is not being able to see them and have them see you. FaceTime, Skype, Webex and Zoom solve that problem. Remember, many COVID -19 patients have to be on a ventilator for at least part of their treatment, which makes them unable to speak. But a video call – quick and easy for any staff member to do – gives both of you the real time contact you need to see each other and to see exactly what's going on.

If you want to use FaceTime or Skype, be sure to write down the user names or passwords you'll need on your Information Central page, so you and the medical staff will have them handy. And don't forget to make sure the app is working on both of your phones before you send your loved one's phone with him to the hospital.

Texting

Is your loved one is awake and able to use his or her phone, but not able to carry on a long conversation? Then texting is a great alternative. The whole family texting little updates, well wishes, pictures, videos and even jokes can really make the day of someone stuck in bed. Texts can also be read back to him once he's awake and able to listen. Some phones like iPhones also let you send an audio or video text which is a great way to send love to or from the hospital or help relieve boredom during recovery.

Social Media

When you have to communicate fast, don't forget Facebook, Twitter and Instagram. They all have instant messaging, so if you need to reach family members quickly, they might just see a direct message faster than a missed call or text.

Games

If your family or friends play group games like Words With Friends online, be sure to tuck this login in your loved ones contacts so they'll have it with them if they want to stay connected. It's a great way to keep some normalcy when everything else seems to be spiraling out of control.

White Board

When you have a chance to talk to the nurses taking care of your loved one, ask them – if they have the time – if they would take a moment to jot down a few updates about your patient on the whiteboard in her room. Any improvements that she's made, what she had for lunch, how they feel her day went. Then when they call to give you an update (preferably twice a day) you won't just get a medical rundown. They'll be able to give you a quick status along with a personal update.

Playlists

If you have time, put together a playlist of power songs, relaxing songs and just plain favorites for your love one to listen to during rough times and recovery. You can also assemble a list of favorite movies that can be streamed along with the name of the streaming service you use, so it's easy for a hospital staff member to help your loved one to find her favorites.

Other Way To Stay In Touch

There is no one more inventive than a family desperate to communicate with someone they love. We've all heard stories the last few weeks of people using walkie-talkies and baby monitors outside their husband's or mom's hospital window to be with them, so they won't be alone.

Some temporary makeshift hospitals might not even have phones at their patient's bedsides. So whatever way you find to stay in communication with sick loved ones – don't ever let anyone – a hospital, doctor, nurse, first responder – anyone – tell you that you won't be able to communicate with the person you love.   You just have to figure out HOW to make it happen.

The most important thing to remember is that the person you love is not alone. You're only a FaceTime (or call or text or Tweet) away.

Vision Board

If you have time, put some paper (poster board or thick drawing paper if you have it), glue, scissors and old magazines in the hospital bag along with your loved one's slippers and toiletries.

Why? So they can create a vision board.

Whether they put one together while their symptoms are mild or once they're beginning to feel better, a vision board is the perfect way to help a sick patient focus on recovery.

The directions are simple. Cut out pictures of what you want to do or to achieve once you recover.

Once it's complete, have the nursing staff post it where the patient can see it. The minute they feel better, have them make a list of exactly how they're going to make all of those things come to pass.

Vision. It's one of the most vital parts of recovery.

How To Put Full ICE Contacts On Your Smartphones

During Hurricane Katrina and the London bombings, so many people were injured, unconscious and separated from their families that a British paramedic, Bob Brotchie came up with the idea of putting ICE Contacts (In Case Of Emergency) on cell phones. Now, when a patient who is unconscious or unable to speak comes into the emergency room, hospitals worldwide check patient's smartphones for an ICE contact, to help them locate their next of kin.

Everyone in your family should have an ICE contact in his or her smartphone. In fact, they should actually have two just in case the first contact is unavailable.   And even if you already have an ICE Contact, that doesn't mean that it has everything in it that it should, to save your life or the life of your spouse or your children.

If you already have an ICE Contact on your phone, don't just skip this section. Take a look at shortcut sheet to make sure your contact has everything it should, before using the instructions to ICE all the other phones in your household.

Since every type of smartphone is different, we have separate instructions on each type of phone.

Just go to the section for your type of phone and let's get started! You'll find instructions for Windows and Non Galaxy Android phones in the downloads.

How To Put An ICE Contact On Your iPhone & Your Apple Medical ID

iPhones are always getting better and Apple's newest effort at keeping customers safe — Medical ID — is amazing. But as much as we LOVE it, there are two reasons you still need to make a regular ICE Contact.

1. You can put an unlimited amount of vital information into a regular contact.

2. Hospitals are used to looking for ICE Contacts rather than Medical ID and if you don't have a regular one, they might miss it.

And with the way the world has been the last few years — remember Hurricane Harvey, Hurricane Irma, Maria and the California Ranch, Camp, Thomas and Carr wildfires — having an ICE contact is an awesome way keep your family safe and connected no matter WHAT is happening around you.

Here's what you'll need:

All of the contact info for your two (or more) emergency contacts.

- A list of your allergies.
- A list of your medical conditions/recent surgeries
- The contact information for your main physician(s)
- Any other information you would like an ER to know about you.

Grab your phone and let's get started!

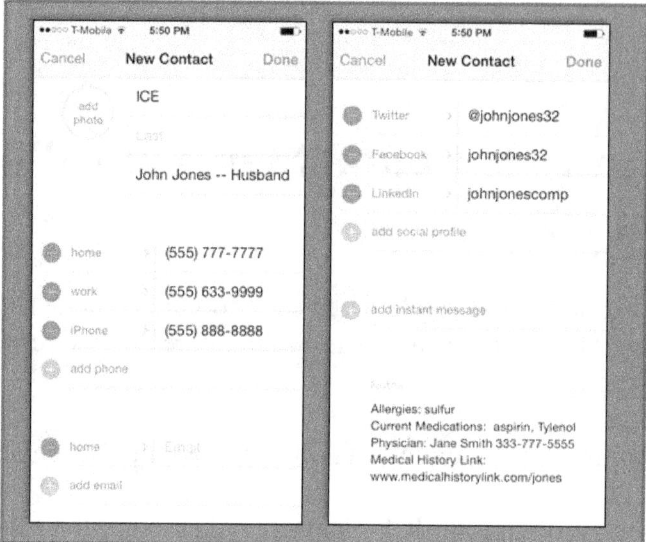

1. Put the word ICE, all capitals, in the First Name field. Don't type anything else in this field!

2. Put your ICE Contact's full name and relationship to you in the Company field, ie John Smith – Husband.

3. Type in every phone number you have for your contact.

4. Type in all of your contact's email addresses — again, every last one.

5. Type in all of your contact's social media handles/user names. You never know what will be up and running in an emergency. Many people have reached loved ones on Facebook and Twitter, when cell phone and landline service was down.

6. All of your own allergies, medications and medical history go in the notes section. Even better capitalize the words ALLERGIES, MEDICATIONS etc to ensure that they're seen.

7. Add your physician's names and phone numbers in the notes section and if you like, a link to your own Medical History Form. You'll find one in this book and in the downloads that came with it.

8. Is your contact in different locations on different days? Add that in the notes section.

9. Instead of their photo, add an ICE Contact Graphic to the contact to make it stand out. Go to the Free Resource Page at http://rnn10.wordpress.com to download your favorite.

10. And finally, never put your social security number or insurance member number into your ICE Contact. You can add the name of your insurance company and customer service number, but the actual numbers can wait until later.

By the way, remember that you can fill in your ICE Contact on your Mac or iPad. Not only is it easier to type on a larger screen, but once you save it to your contacts, it will sync with iCloud and appear right on your phone.

And now, let's make your ICE info even easier to find, by setting up your iPhone's Medical ID.

What Is Medical ID?

Medical ID, a part of the Apple Health App, not only gives you a place to put your emergency medical information, but it puts a link to that information right on the front of your phone, where it can be viewed by a hospital even if your phone is password locked.

You'll find it on most iPhones (iPhone 6 and up) using iOS 8 and higher.   If your phone is older and doesn't have Medical ID, you can just leave your ICE Contact the way it is.

On your home screen click on the Health App – it's the one with the heart on it. This will take you to the Dashboard page of the Health App. On the bottom right of the screen, you'll see the Medical ID icon. Click on it.

On the Medical ID screen, click on the red link that says Create Medical ID.

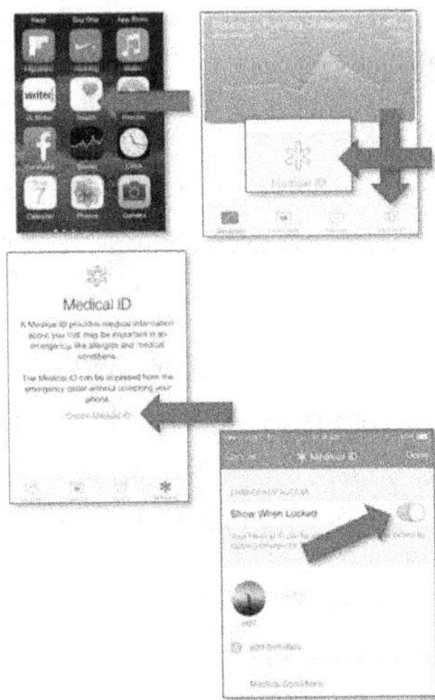

The most important part of the Medical ID screen is at the top. It's the On/Off Switch that shows a link to your emergency information on the home screen of your phone even when it's password-locked.

Before you do anything else, switch this to the ON position. It will turn green like the graphic below.

By the way, none of the information in your Medical ID is shared with any of the other apps on your phone.

Enter All Of Your Information

Put all the information you possibly can into your Medical ID.

As you can see it already has fields for your birth date, medical conditions, allergies, current medications and other information. There are two sections that you need to pay special attention to – Medical Notes and Add Emergency Contact.

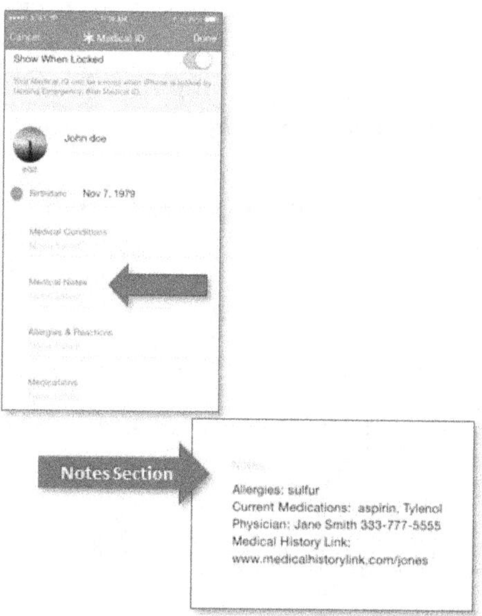

After you finish filling in the regular fields, use the Notes Section to list anything that didn't fit into them, like the names and phone numbers of your physicians and healthcare providers and contact information for your Insurance Company. Again, don't add any sensitive personal information like a social security number, insurance member ID number or financial information.

You can also place a link to your Medical History Form in the Notes Section to give emergency personnel to quick access to your medical history until your emergency contact arrives at the hospital.

Add Your Emergency Contact

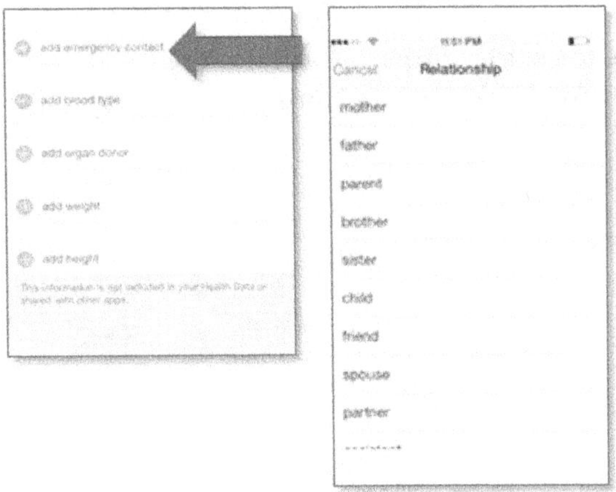

When you click on Medical ID's Add Emergency Contact button, it will show you a list of your contacts, so you can choose the people you'd like to add to your Medical ID. That's why we had you set up your ICE Contacts first.

Go ahead and click on the button and choose your first ICE Contact.

If you have additional ICE Contacts (a smart idea, in case your first contact is unreachable), then click on the Add Emergency Contact field again to add as many additional people as you would like.

Want to save time turning your husband or wife's contact into an ICE Contact? Simple! Just tap & hold the contact you want to use, choose share and email it to yourself. Then open it in your email, make the changes from above to turn it into an ICE Contact and save it to your contacts as ICE.
That's all there is to it!

And don't forget to put ICE Contacts on your spouse's and kid's phones too, along with each other's contact information, so you can all get in touch with each other quickly in an emergency.

Having an ICE contact and Medical ID is an awesome way keep your family safe and connected no matter WHAT is happening around you.

MEET THE WHOLE FAMILY

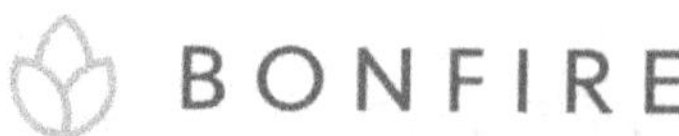

A percentage of each product sold will go towards putting our newest book *#Alone Together*, into the hands of the families who need it. The book's mission? To help keep hospitalized COVID-19 patients from dying alone, by giving their families the tools they need to stay connected with them and their medical team.

To purchase masks, mugs & tee shirts   https://www.bonfire.com/store/getyourstufftogether/
To purchase phone cases   https://www.zazzle.com/s/wealthoftulips+phone+cases

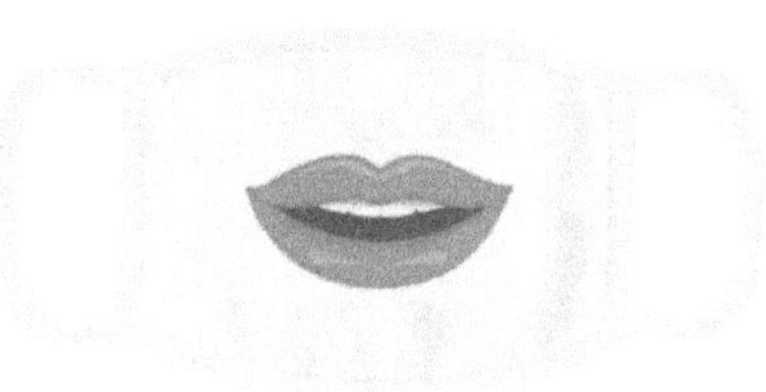

Richly Red Smile Mask

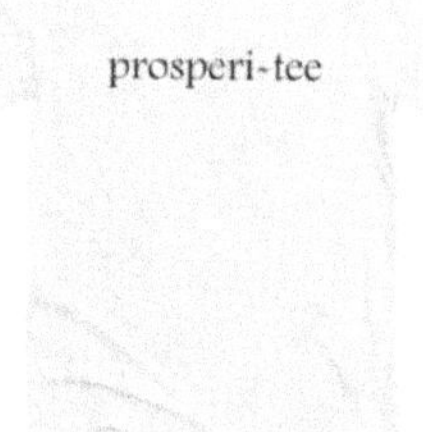

Creativi-Tea Coffee &Tea Mug

Prosperi-Tee Tee Shirt

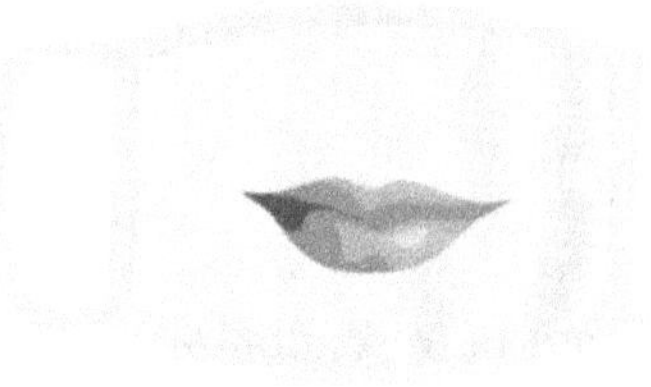

Pretty In Pink Smile Mask

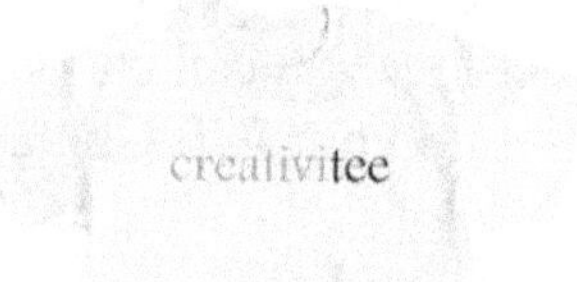

Leftea Coffee &Tea Mug

Creativi-Tee Tee Shirt

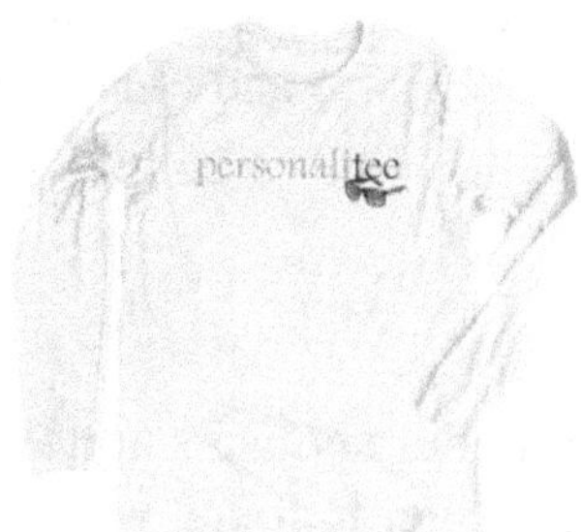

Red Parrot Tulip Phone Case

Personali-Tee Tee Shirt

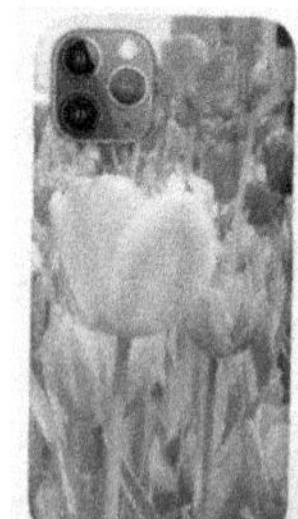
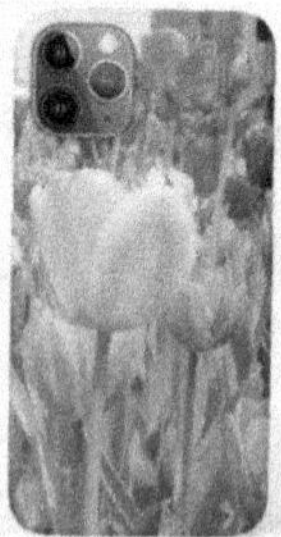

Tulips In Breeze Phone Case

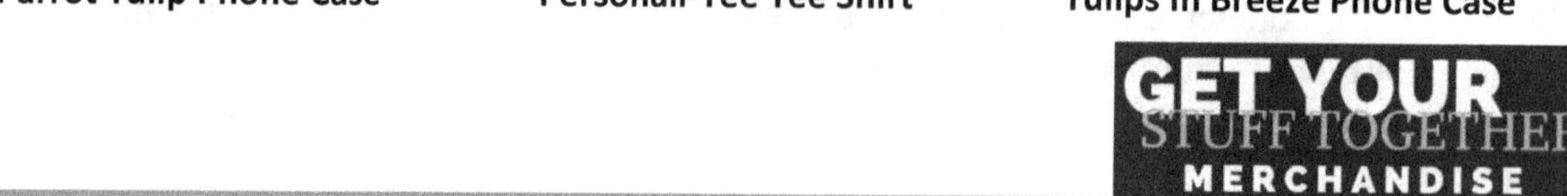

How To Put An ICE Contact On Your Samsung Galaxy

What Is iCE?

During Hurricane Katrina, so many people were injured & separated from their families, that emergency workers came up with the idea of putting an iCE – In Case Of Emergency – contact in their cell phones. Now, hospitals worldwide, check patient's phones for their iCE contact, to locate their next of kin.

Everyone in your family should have 2 iCE contacts on his cell phone, just in case the first person is unavailable. So let's learn how to set up your iCE contact on your Samsung Galaxy.

Grab Your Phone & Let's Get Started 1

Who will your two iCE Contacts be? Your spouse, partner, best friend, parent or close relative? Once you decide, **Touch** the **Contacts Icon** on your Galaxy to open up your Contacts. Click on the plus sign + to add a new contact and **touch the First Name Field.** Don't put the name of your contact in this field, only the word **iCE.** This is because your Galaxy sorts contacts by their first name by default.

Next, touch the **Last Name Field** and enter your contact's full name, ie. John Jones. Now when someone looks at the contact, they'll see iCE along with your emergency contact's full name.   Do the same thing for your second iCE contact – just call it ICE2.

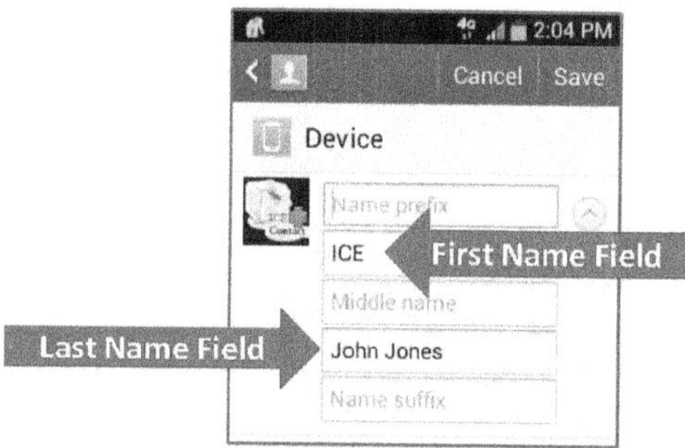

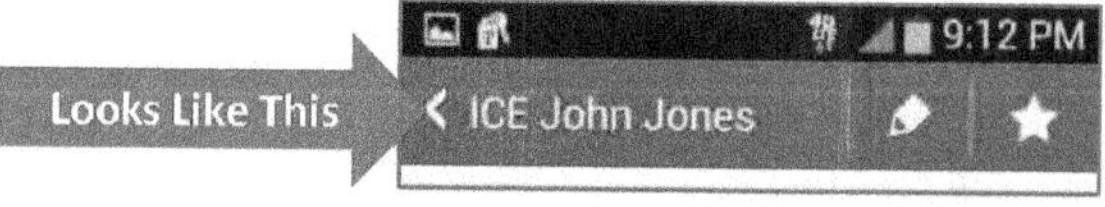

Enter All of Your Information 2

Put **all the information you possibly can** into your two iCE Contacts. For example:
- Your emergency contact's **Main Number/Cell number/ Work number, Relationship** to you
- **Email Address & IM, Twitter and Facebook** address (in case landlines are down & you need to send an emergency message)
- Other info, for example, days that the contact is at a certain location
- Add **extra fields** if you need them.
- Use the **Notes Section** to list your Allergies, Current Medications or the Names & Numbers of your Physicians.

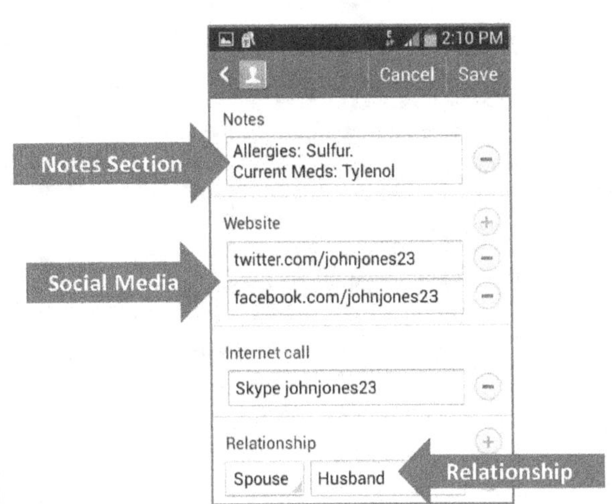

Adding Fields 3

To add fields to your contact, press and hold the field name until the menu appears, then check the boxes next to the field/label you want and clicking OK.

One great field to add is **Relationship**, to tell emergency personnel who your contact is to you.

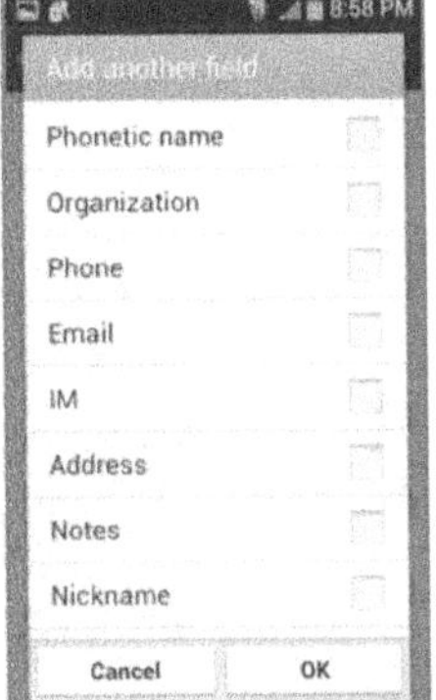

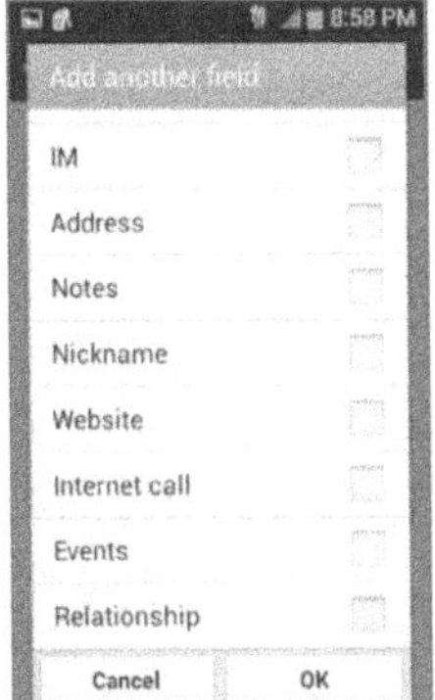

What About Your Medical History? 4

Need more than just a few lines to communicate your medical history? Then create a medical history form and store it to a password protected online folder & place a link to the form in your iCE contact. This way a doctor can access your, your spouse's or your kids basic medical history, while you're en route to the hospital.   You'll find your Medical Information Forms in the materials you downloaded at the beginning of the book and a Shortcut Sheet in the chapter on Medical History.

By the way, don't forget to make emergency cards for you and your family too. You'll find instructions later in this book.

Make Your iCE Contacts Stand Out

5

Make your iCE contacts stand out, by using the **Add Photo** function to upload a graphic to your phone, like the ones on this page. You can make your own, or use ours. You'll find them with the Forms you downloaded at the beginning of the book. Save the graphic to the photos on your phone. Open your ICE Contact, **Touch** the little photo icon, **Choose Image**, pick the graphic you want and **Save**.

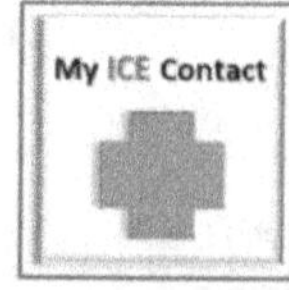

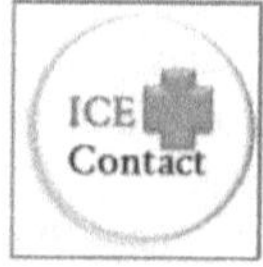

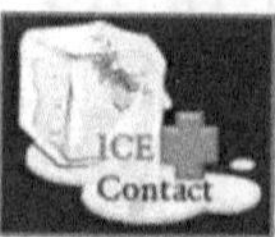

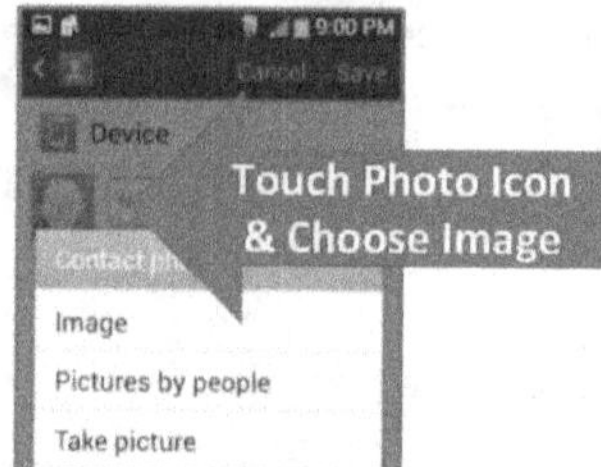

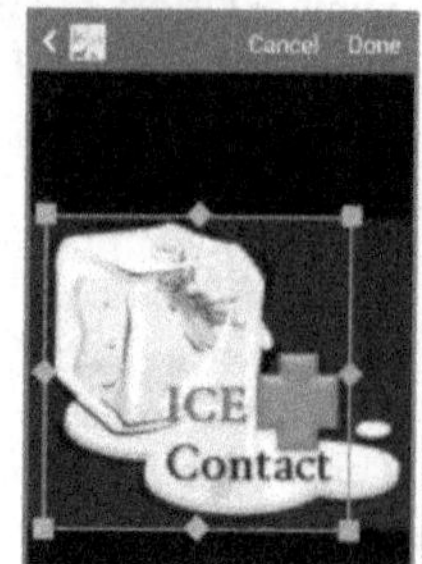

What If You Password Lock Your Galaxy?

6

If you lock your phone with a password, it would be difficult for emergency personnel to retrieve your **ICE Contact**. But don't worry. There are 2 ways around that.

Most Samsung Galaxies have an **Emergency Dialer** on the **Home Screen**. Simply set up your ICE contacts and then press and hold your first ICE contact until the menu appears, then add it to the **ICE Emergency Contact Group**. Now it will appear on your emergency dialer.

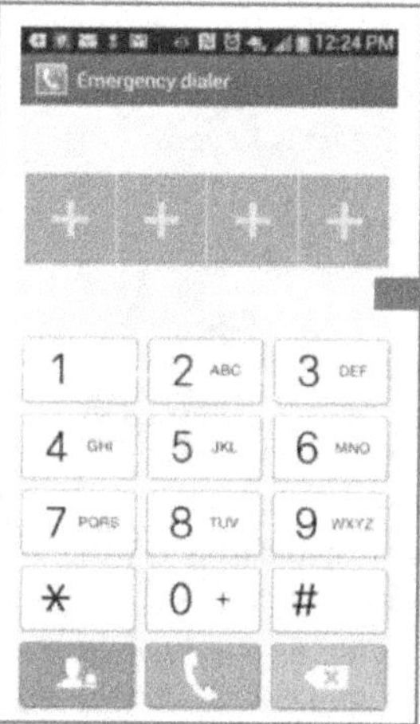

Phone	Groups	Favorites	Contacts
Not assigned			(10)
Integrated groups			
ICE - emergency contacts			(1)
Co-workers			(0)
Family			(0)
Friends			(0)

What If You Don't Have Emergency Dialer? 7

If your Galaxy doesn't have this feature, but you normally password lock your phone, all you have to do is add your ICE information directly to your **Lock Screen**. Here's how you do it:

Go into **Settings** and touch **My Device** and then **Lock Screen**. Then touch **Lock Screen Widgets**. Now on the very bottom of the menu you'll see **Owner Information**. Touch that and a window will appear. Simply type in "ICE CONTACT" along with your contact's name, phone number, your allergy or medical information – anything you would need an emergency room to know about you.   Then **Check the Box** and Choose **Okay**.

Now your ICE information will appear right on your Lock Screen, no password needed.

Problem solved!

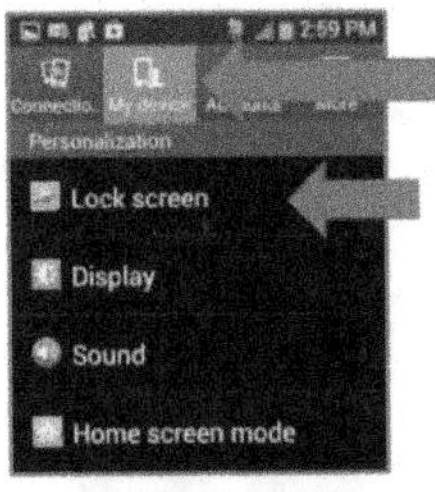

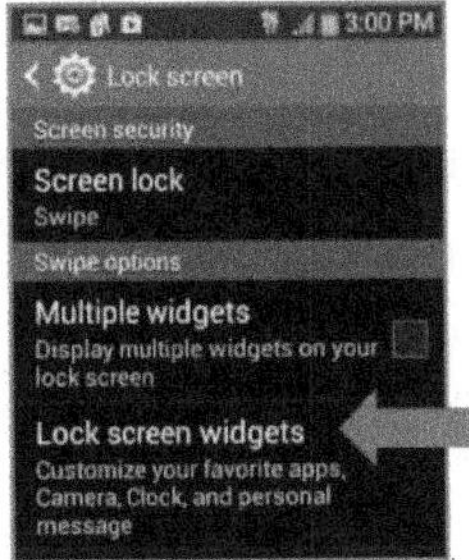

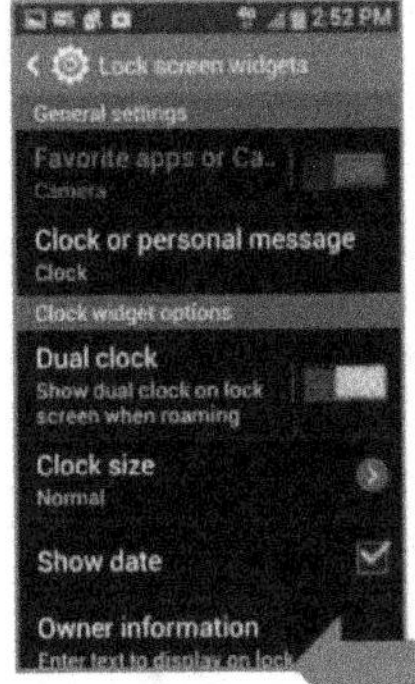

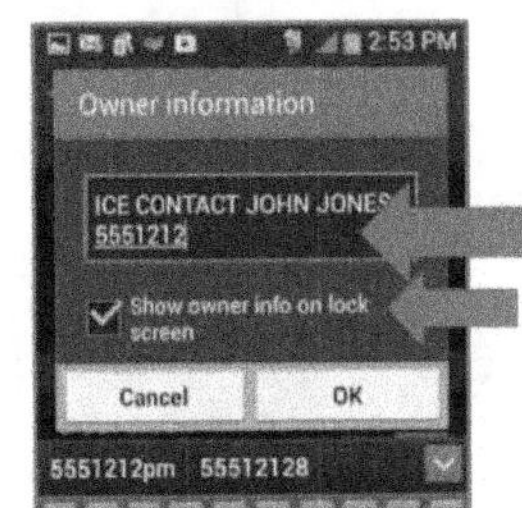

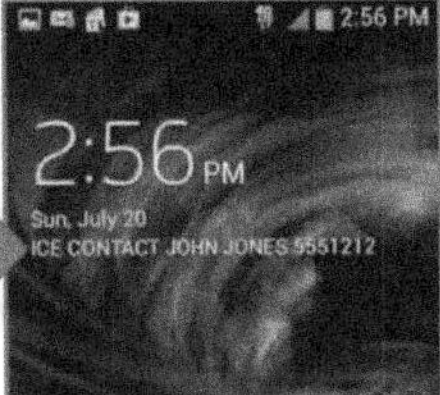

Turn Your Phone Into A Mobile Command Center 8

While you're at it, you can even **turn your phone** into a **Mobile Command Center**. Just store copies of your family's medical history forms, emergency action plans, checklists and Evacuation Plan (which you can find in our book The Backup Plan 3.0), right on your phone and the phones of each member of your immediate family.

And don't forget to put iCE Contacts on their phones as well.

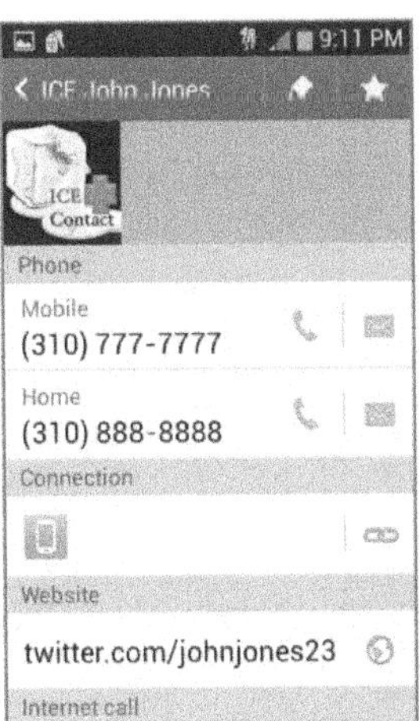

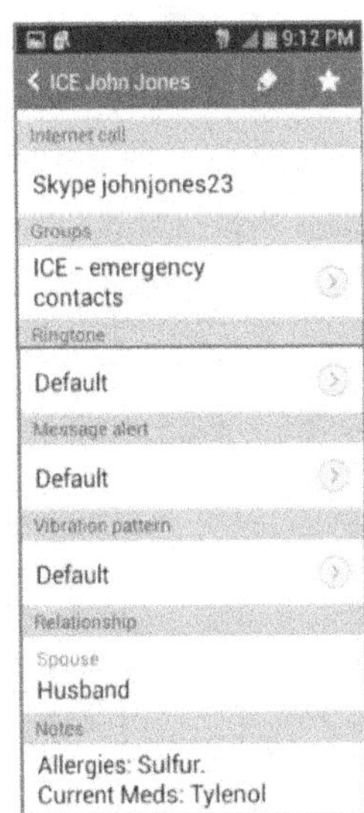

How To Put An ICE Contact On Your Older Cell Phone

What Is iCE?

During Hurricane Katrina, so many people were injured & separated from their families, that emergency workers came up with the idea of putting an iCE – In Case Of Emergency – contact in their cell phones. Now, hospitals worldwide, check patient's phones for their iCE contact, to locate their next of kin.   Everyone in your family should have 2 iCE contacts on his cell phone, just in case the first person is unavailable.

These instructions are for regular cell phones – not smartphones. But don't worry. Even if your phone isn't a smartphone, it's just as easy to set up an ICE Contact. Just keep in mind that every phone is different, so you might have to play around with the contact a bit, to get all the information you want to include.

Grab Your Phone & Let's Get Started

1

Who will your two iCE Contacts be? Your spouse, partner, best friend, parent or close relative? Once you decide, **Touch** the **Contacts Icon** on your phone to open up your Contacts.

Depending on the type of phone you have, your Contacts Icon might look different than the ones we have here. Click on **Add New** to add a new contact and **touch the First Name Field.** Don't put the name of your contact in this field, only the word **iCE.**

Next, touch the **Last Name Field** and enter your contact's full name and relationship to you, ie. John Jones Husband. Now when someone looks at the contact, they'll see ICE along with your emergency contact's full name.   Do the same thing for your second iCE contact – just call it ICE2.

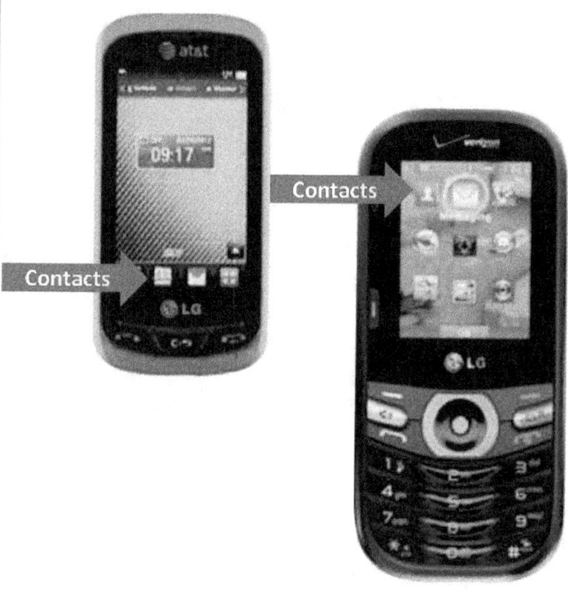

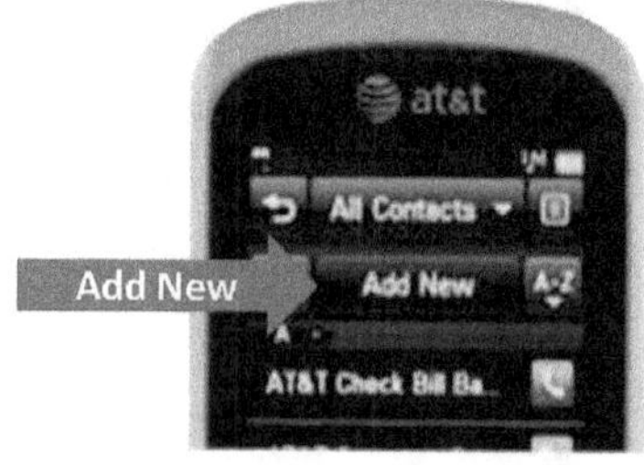

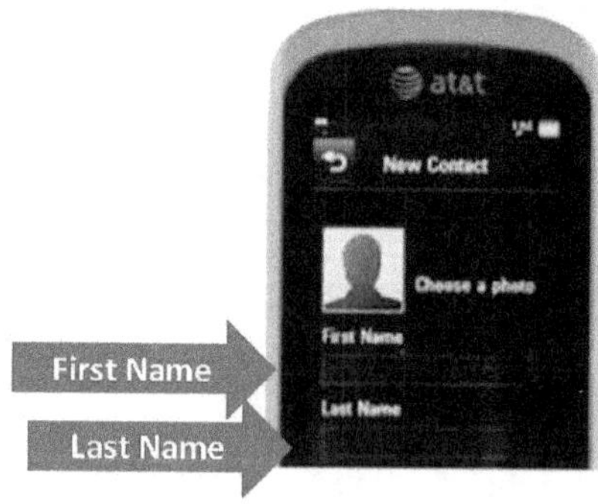

Enter All of The Information You Can   2

Put **all the information you possibly can** into your two iCE Contacts. For example:
- Your emergency contact's **Main Number/Cell number/ Work number**
- **Email Address & Social Media Contacts** like their **Facebook** address (in case landlines are down & emergency personnel need to send an emergency message)
- Other info, for example, days that the contact is at a certain location
- If you have a section for Notes in your contact, use the **Notes Section** to list your Allergies, Medications or Doctor's Contact Information.

What About Your Medical History?   3

Need more than just a few lines to communicate your medical history? Then create a medical history form and store it to a password protected online folder & place a link to the form in your iCE contact. This way a doctor can access your, your spouse's or your kids basic medical history, while you're en route to the hospital.   You'll find your Medical Information Forms in the materials you downloaded at the beginning of the book and a Shortcut Sheet in the chapter on Medical History.

By the way, don't forget to make emergency cards for you and your family too. You'll find instructions later in this book.

Make Your iCE Contacts Stand Out   4

Make your iCE contacts stand out, by using the **Add Photo** function to upload a graphic to your phone, like the ones on this page.

Not every cell phone has the ability to do this, but if you can add a picture to a contact, you should be able to add one of our graphics, instead.

You'll find them with the Forms you downloaded at the beginning of the book. First, save the graphic to the photos on your phone. Since you're not working with a smartphone, you might have to email the graphic to yourself from your computer or even take a picture of the graphic you'd like to use, with your phone. Once you get it into your photos folder on your phone, open your ICE Contact, **Touch** the little photo icon, go into your photos, choose your graphic and **Save**.

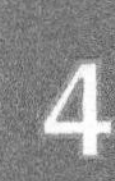

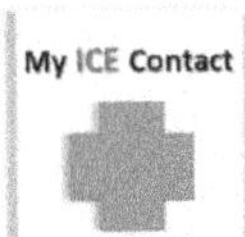

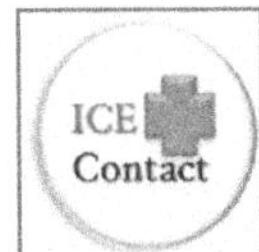

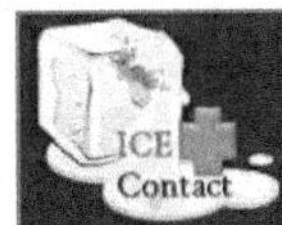

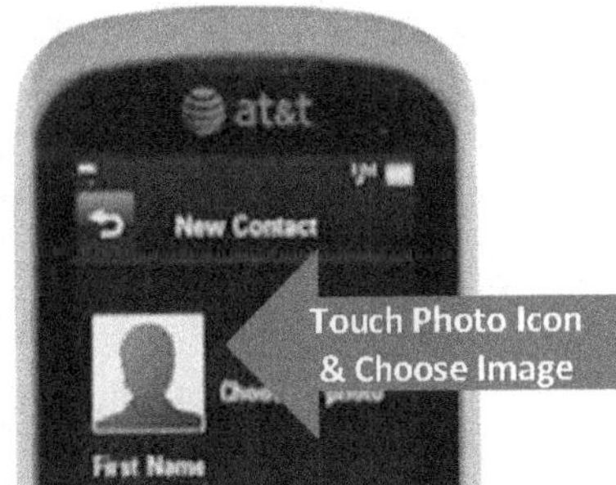

The Smart Contact©

An ICE Contact can be a real lifesaver, especially in an emergency, when an ER doctor can use it to learn everything she needs to know about your medical history in one minute flat.

But thankfully life-threatening emergencies don't happen every day. What DOES happen, is that moms, dads and caregivers need to have important details about their children, their parents and the people they care for, at their fingertips.

Whether you're at the doctor, registering for school, visiting a specialist, or sitting in the emergency room with a slightly dented child, you never know when you're going to need potentially lifesaving details for the people you love.

That's why we re-engineered the entire concept of the ICE Contact, by turning it on its head.

Meet the Smart Contact$^{©}$ – the contact that gives you all of the information you need, right in your smartphone. Not only will it come in handy in any of the situations we mentioned above, but it also contains all of the contact information you need to locate and gather your family members in minutes.

Simply create one Smart Contact$^{©}$ for each member of your immediate family and if necessary, your parents and adult children. You probably already have a contact on your phone for many of these people, so simply add the information on the shortcut sheet below to their existing contact, to transform it into the perfect Smart Contact$^{©}$.

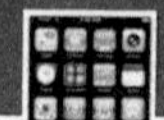

Your Mission, Should You Choose To Accept It...

...is to set up a Smart Contact for each member of your immediate family, including your parents, adult children and any people for which you provide care. Since you already have a contact on your phone for most of these people, just add the information on the shortcut sheet below, to their contacts for an instant Smart Contact.

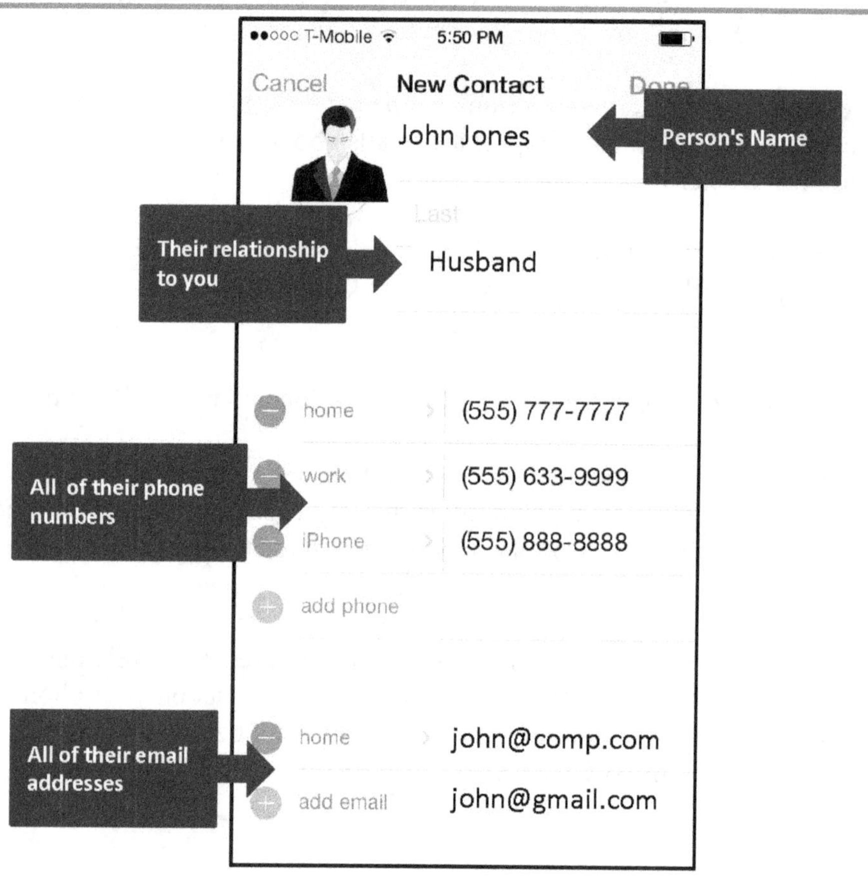

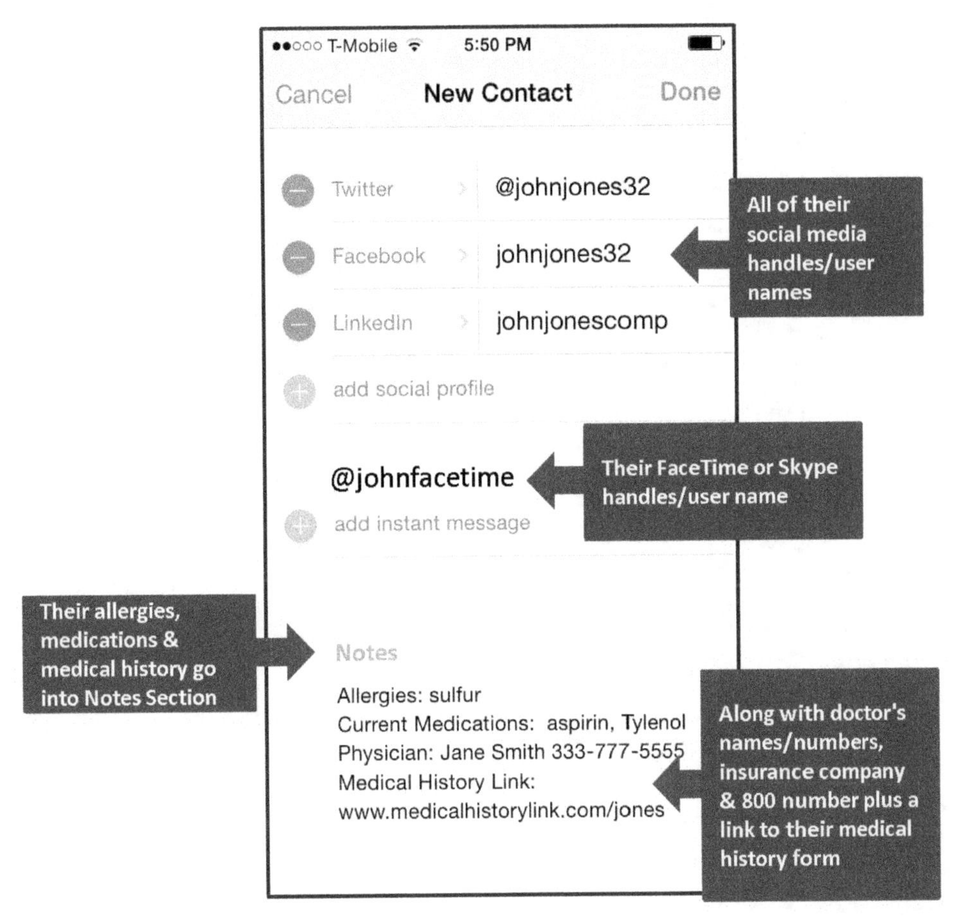

All of their social media handles/user names

Their FaceTime or Skype handles/user name

Their allergies, medications & medical history go into Notes Section

Along with doctor's names/numbers, insurance company & 800 number plus a link to their medical history form

Online, Social Media & Business Passwords

Many of the people who have COVID-19 haven't been able to communicate for at least part of the time that they're hospitalized.   And chances are good their spouse, parent or children might have to handle something for them while they're sick.

I had a good friend who set up a separate bank account to collect the money that he made from selling an online book. I was there when he set it up, so when he passed away unexpectedly, I was able to tell his wife that she needed to find the account and change it to her name. He didn't remember to write down the logins or information about the account, so if I wouldn't have been able to tell her about it, she never would have found that money.

That's why we've included a copy of our book Online in your download. It comes with all of the forms that you need to keep your social media account information at your fingertips, in a digital format. Just open the forms, fill them in and save them to your computer or print them out.

This way if you need a copy of your social media or online logons quickly, you can retrieve them from any Internet-enabled computer, cellphone or tablet, enabling you to deal with emergencies large and small.

There are three parts to the book. The first section is for your personal logins, passwords and URLs and the second, for your business. If you need more space, just add lines to the downloadable documents or print out the forms and put them into a notebook.

The third section is called a **Social Media Will**. Not that you will EVER need it, but it is a place to jot down how you or your loved one would want their websites, social media accounts and internet accounts handled if they were incapacitated or suddenly passed away.

Once you've completed the My Social Life forms and Social Media Will for each adult member of your family, we suggest that you print them out to have them at your fingertips during the pandemic and then afterwards, save and store them in at least three secure locations.

How To Make Your Family Findable

Living In A State of Constant Communication

In the middle of a busy, but quiet day in a Midwestern university lecture hall, the silence was pierced by a sudden hail of gunfire. Students ran out of the hall and ducked under tables. Those who couldn't move tried to make themselves as invisible as possible until help arrived. That day at Northern Illinois University, five students lost their lives. Many others were injured.

As the police and security were struggling to control the situation, a number of the student's parents not only knew that their children were all right, but they knew exactly what was happening in real time.

So how did some people have a window into the NIU tragedy while others did not? Facebook and Twitter! As unlikely as it sounds, students ingeniously found a way to use their favorite method of keeping in touch with friends, as a tool to connect to the outside world in the middle of a crisis.

Students caught under desks and tables grabbed their smartphones and started communicating. Tweets went out on Twitter, notes and messages went up on Facebook pages, telling friends and family that students, who were literally in the thick of things, were all right.

Others told loved ones or security officers the location of trapped students, facilitating their rescue. Friends started texting each other to find out where everyone was and, in the hours that followed, created Facebook pages memorializing the fallen.

It was an amazing display of people, who are connected 24/7, using that same technology to communicate, connect, survive and heal.

During the Japan earthquake cell phone towers barely worked because of earthquake damage and overloaded networks. But Wi-Fi was up and running. So what kept the Japanese connected with their families and the outside world? Twitter, Facebook, Skype and YouTube!

Smartphones, tablets and notebook computers are a phenomenal way to stay in touch during an emergency. Whether you send an email, text, tweet or Facebook message, you can find out the location and condition of everyone you love in seconds.   In a dire emergency, you can even send help, confirm or update emergency plans and even mobilize family and friends to be at the side of the ill or injured, using real time information.

Since disasters are completely unpredictable, the only way to prepare yourself and your family is to give yourselves as many different avenues of communication as possible.   You never know which one will make the difference.

Want to learn how your family can use technology to communicate during an emergency? Then let's get started.

Your Mission, Should You Choose To Accept It...

...is to learn how your family can use technology to communicate during an emergency, then create a smartphone based communication plan to use the next time you have to gather everybody in a hurry.

Updating Your Smartphones — 1

When you created your Family Evacuation Plan (if you haven't done that yet, go do it now – we'll wait for you), you listed the phone numbers, email addresses and social media addresses for each family member in your household.

Now we're going to take that one step further by adding all of that information to each family member's smartphones. While you're at it, add new contacts on everyone's phones for all of your out-of-area emergency contacts as well.

When Time Is An Issue — 3

Using a social media platform like HootSuite.com may help. With HootSuite, you can send a single message that can be posted to Twitter, Facebook and LinkedIn simultaneously, ensuring that your family or friends would see your message immediately, no matter what site they happen to be on at the moment.

Direct Messaging — 2

If cell phone service is down and you are unable to text, don't forget that Twitter and Facebook can also be used to send direct messages - personal messages that go only to the recipient . Here's a quick tutorial.

First, you need to make sure that every member of your family is following or has "liked" all of the other family members on Twitter and Facebook, so you can direct message each other.

- For Twitter, click on Messages, then Direct Messages and then type in @ and the family member's username. Then type in your message and hit send.
- For Facebook, click the little message icon at the top of your page (between the little people and the little earth). Then click Send New Message and type in the name of the recipient or recipients and click send.

The Value Of A Photo — 4

During the Joplin tornado, even lifelong residents found themselves disoriented when the tornado turned their normal landmarks into kindling. If your spouse or kids don't know where they are after an emergency and need help a quick photo texted or uploaded to Instagram or Facebook could help you locate them. This is especially true of GPS enabled phones or photos with geo-location.

Creating A Communications Plan — 5

Once you and your family have updated your phones and completed your evacuation plans, sit down with them to discuss the ways you can use technology to stay in touch with each other during a disaster.

Come up with some sample scenarios; for example, if a disaster were to happen while your family members were at work, at school or running errands during a normal day.

- How would you connect with each other?
- Would you text each other, or would calling or emailing be faster?
- If you have teens or young adults at home, their natural proclivity may be to send out a text or a tweet on Twitter, to update everyone, including you, on their location or situation.
- Find out the types of communication everyone prefers and then create an emergency communication plan that makes sense for your family.

Grab The Sat Phone! — 7

If you're in an area with frequent emergencies like tornadoes or hurricanes, live out in the country or have a family member in a foreign country, consider getting satellite phones.

They work in remote areas where there is no cell phone coverage and when cell towers are down. Our favorite satellite phone provider is **Iridium**. They have a wide range of satellite phones as well as Iridium Go! Which provides global voice calling and text messaging solutions for your smartphone.

What If... — 6

Another great discussion to have with your family, especially with school age children, is what they would do if they had to get a hold of you but the cell phone system was out, or what to do if there was an area-wide blackout. Don't laugh, that actually happed to us in California!

Kids are so used to technology that they might not have the experience that they need to do things the old school way. The best way to plan is to give yourselves as many ways as possible to stay connected. Then if one or two normal methods are unusable, you'll all simply turn to a different method to reach each other.

Code Word Clearance Or Higher — 8

Consider creating a Family Emergency Code or Code Word. This is a code or word that only you and your immediate family know. When a family member says it, texts it or emails it to the rest of the family, it signals that they're in trouble and need help.

It's only to be used in extreme emergency and means that everyone needs to drop what they're doing and establish contact with each other, immediately.

Find My Family ASAP! — 9

Find My Friends is an iPhone app that is designed to let you know at a glance where your friends are. But you can also use it to immediately locate your children, spouse and loved ones in an emergency.

All your family has to do is allow you access on their phones, and if need be, you can immediately see where everyone is in real time, complete with map and directions.

Medical Information Forms & Emergency Wallet Cards

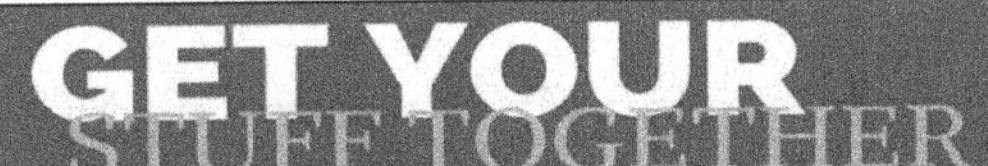

Adult One - Medical

Section One — Adult One Information

First Name	MI	Last Name	M/F	DOB

Religion	Home Phone	Cell Phone	Work Phone	Email Address

Address	City	State	Zip

Height/Weight	Blood Type	RH	Identifying Marks

Section Two — Emergency Contacts

Main Contact:

First Name	Last Name	Relationship	Home Phone	Work Phone	Cell

Best Place to Reach Contact? Any Schedule Considerations? Notes?

Contact Two

First Name	Last Name	Relationship	Home Phone	Work Phone	Cell

Best Place to Reach Contact? Any Schedule Considerations? Notes?

Contact Three

First Name	Last Name	Relationship	Home Phone	Work Phone	Cell

Best Place to Reach Contact? Any Schedule Considerations? Notes?

Work

Employer	Title	Phone	Manager

Address	City	State	Zip

Section Three — Medical Information

Primary Physician	Specialty	Phone	Alt Phone/Email	Hospital
Physician Two	Specialty	Phone	Alt Phone/Email	Hospital
Physician Three	Specialty	Phone	Alt Phone/Email	Hospital

Dentist	Specialty	Phone	Alt Phone/Email	Notes

Dentist Two	Specialty	Phone	Alt Phone/Email	Notes

Optometrist	Glasses/Contacts?	Phone	Alt Phone/Email	Location

Section Four — Prescription, Allergy & Chronic Condition Information

Prescription Information

Prescription Name	Dosage	Frequency	For what condition
Prescription Name	Dosage	Frequency	For what condition
Prescription Name	Dosage	Frequency	For what condition
Prescription Name	Dosage	Frequency	For what condition

Name of Pharmacy	Phone	Pharmacist	Location

Allergy Information

Allergy Type	Severity	Frequency/Last Occurrence/Notes
Allergy Type	Severity	Frequency/Last Occurrence/Notes
Allergy Type	Severity	Frequency/Last Occurrence/Notes

Chronic Conditions

Condition	Severity	Current Treatment/Notes
Condition	Severity	Current Treatment/Notes
Condition	Severity	Current Treatment/Notes

Immunizations

Immunization	Date	Immunization	Date
Immunization	Date	Immunization	Date
Immunization	Date	Immunization	Date

Section Five — Health Insurance

Insurance Company	Member Number	Group/Policy Number	Customer Service

Member Hospital	Agent Name	Agent Number	Notes

Insurance Company	Member Number	Group/Policy Number	Customer Service

Member Hospital	Agent Name	Agent Number	Notes

Section Six — Do You Have A….

Will?	Location	Power of Attorney?	Location
Living Will/Trust?	Location	Other	Location

Section Seven — Important Things To Know

Things I want an emergency physician to know about me

Things I want an emergency physician to know about my medical history

Any other notes, important numbers or wishes that need to be communicated

Section Eight — Recent Medical Procedures and Tests

Procedure 1	Date	Reason for Procedure
Physician	Hospital	Results
Procedure 2	Date	Reason for Procedure
Physician	Hospital	Results
Medical Test 1	Date	Reason for Procedure
Physician	Hospital	Results
Medical Test 2	Date	Reason for Procedure
Physician	Hospital	Results
Medical Test 3	Date	Reason for Procedure
Physician	Hospital	Results

Section Nine — Alternative Medicines and Other Substances Commonly Used

Vitamins or Herbs Taken	Dosage	Frequency/Last Occurrence/Notes

itamins or Herbs Taken	Dosage	Frequency/Last Occurrence/Notes

Vitamins or Herbs Taken	Dosage	Frequency/Last Occurrence/Notes

Substances or Alcohol Used	Frequency	Substances or Alcohol Used	Frequency
Substances or Alcohol Used	Frequency	Substances or Alcohol Used	Frequency
Substances or Alcohol Used	Frequency	Substances or Alcohol Used	Frequency

Section Ten	Counselors or Other Health Providers		
Counselor 1	Specialty	Phone	Alternate Phone
Counselor 2	Specialty	Phone	Alternate Phone

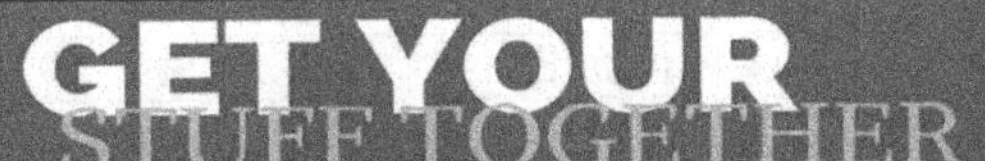

Adult Two - Medical

Section One — Adult One Information

First Name	MI	Last Name		M/F	DOB

Religion	Home Phone	Cell Phone		Work Phone	Email Address

Address		City		State	Zip

Height/Weight	Blood Type	RH		Identifying Marks	

Section Two — Emergency Contacts

Main Contact:

First Name	Last Name	Relationship	Home Phone	Work Phone	Cell

Best Place to Reach Contact? Any Schedule Considerations? Notes?

Contact Two

First Name	Last Name	Relationship	Home Phone	Work Phone	Cell

Best Place to Reach Contact? Any Schedule Considerations? Notes?

Contact Three

First Name	Last Name	Relationship	Home Phone	Work Phone	Cell

Best Place to Reach Contact? Any Schedule Considerations? Notes?

Work

Employer	Title	Phone	Manager

Address	City	State	Zip

Section Three — Medical Information

Primary Physician	Specialty	Phone	Alt Phone/Email	Hospital

Physician Two	Specialty	Phone	Alt Phone/Email	Hospital

Physician Three	Specialty	Phone	Alt Phone/Email	Hospital

Dentist	Specialty	Phone	Alt Phone/Email	Notes

Dentist Two	Specialty	Phone	Alt Phone/Email	Notes

Optometrist	Glasses/Contacts?	Phone	Alt Phone/Email	Location

Section Four — Prescription, Allergy & Chronic Condition Information

Prescription Information

Prescription Name	Dosage	Frequency	For what condition
Prescription Name	Dosage	Frequency	For what condition
Prescription Name	Dosage	Frequency	For what condition
Prescription Name	Dosage	Frequency	For what condition

Name of Pharmacy	Phone	Pharmacist	Location

Allergy Information

Allergy Type	Severity	Frequency/Last Occurrence/Notes
Allergy Type	Severity	Frequency/Last Occurrence/Notes
Allergy Type	Severity	Frequency/Last Occurrence/Notes

Chronic Conditions

Condition	Severity	Current Treatment/Notes
Condition	Severity	Current Treatment/Notes
Condition	Severity	Current Treatment/Notes

Immunizations

Immunization	Date	Immunization	Date
Immunization	Date	Immunization	Date
Immunization	Date	Immunization	Date

Section Five — Health Insurance

Insurance Company	Member Number	Group/Policy Number	Customer Service

Member Hospital	Agent Name	Agent Number	Notes

Insurance Company	Member Number	Group/Policy Number	Customer Service

Member Hospital	Agent Name	Agent Number	Notes

Section Six — Do You Have A….

Will?	Location	Power of Attorney?	Location
Living Will/Trust?	Location	Other	Location

Section Seven — Important Things To Know

Things I want an emergency physician to know about me

Things I want an emergency physician to know about my medical history

Any other notes, important numbers or wishes that need to be communicated

Section Eight — Recent Medical Procedures and Tests

Procedure 1	Date	Reason for Procedure
Physician	Hospital	Results
Procedure 2	Date	Reason for Procedure
Physician	Hospital	Results
Medical Test 1	Date	Reason for Procedure
Physician	Hospital	Results
Medical Test 2	Date	Reason for Procedure
Physician	Hospital	Results
Medical Test 3	Date	Reason for Procedure
Physician	Hospital	Results

Section Nine — Alternative Medicines and Other Substances Commonly Used

Vitamins or Herbs Taken	Dosage	Frequency/Last Occurrence/Notes

Vitamins or Herbs Taken		Dosage		Frequency/Last Occurrence/Notes	
Vitamins or Herbs Taken		Dosage		Frequency/Last Occurrence/Notes	
Substances or Alcohol Used	Frequency		Substances or Alcohol Used	Frequency	
Substances or Alcohol Used	Frequency		Substances or Alcohol Used	Frequency	
Substances or Alcohol Used	Frequency		Substances or Alcohol Used	Frequency	

Section Ten	Counselors or Other Health Providers			
Counselor 1	Specialty	Phone	Alternate Phone	
Counselor 2	Specialty	Phone	Alternate Phone	

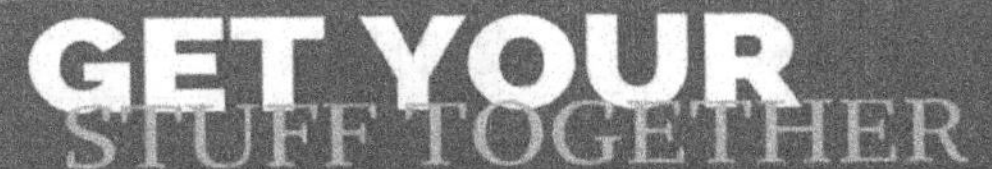

Child - Medical

Section One — Child One Information

First Name	MI	Last Name	M/F	DOB

Religion	Home Phone	Cell Phone	Notes

Address	City	State	Zip

Height/Weight	Blood Type	RH	Identifying Marks

Section Two — Emergency Contacts

Parent/Guardian One:

First Name	Last Name	Relationship	Home Phone	Work Phone	Cell Phone

Best Place to Reach Contact? Any Schedule Considerations? Notes?

Parent/Guardian Two:

First Name	Last Name	Relationship	Home Phone	Work Phone	Cell Phone

Best Place to Reach Contact? Any Schedule Considerations? Notes?

Contact Three

First Name	Last Name	Relationship	Home Phone	Work Phone	Cell Phone

Best Place to Reach Contact? Any Schedule Considerations? Notes?

School

School	Phone	Teacher	Grade

Address	City	Notes

Babysitter	Phone	Afterschool Program #	Phone

Section Three — Medical Information

Primary Pediatrician	Specialty	Phone	Alt Phone/Email	Hospital

Physician Two	Specialty	Phone	Alt Phone/Email	Hospital

Dentist	Specialty	Phone	Alt Phone/Email	Notes

Optometrist	Glasses/Contacts?	Phone	Alt Phone/Email	Location

Section Four		**Prescription, Allergy & Chronic Condition Information**	

Prescription Information

Prescription Name	Dosage	Frequency	For what condition
Prescription Name	Dosage	Frequency	For what condition
Prescription Name	Dosage	Frequency	For what condition
Prescription Name	Dosage	Frequency	For what condition
Name of Pharmacy	Phone	Pharmacist	Location

Allergy Information

Allergy Type	Severity	Frequency/Last Occurrence/Notes
Allergy Type	Severity	Frequency/Last Occurrence/Notes
Allergy Type	Severity	Frequency/Last Occurrence/Notes

Chronic Conditions

Condition	Severity	Current Treatment/Notes
Condition	Severity	Current Treatment/Notes

Immunizations

Immunization	Date	Immunization	Date
Immunization	Date	Immunization	Date
Immunization	Date	Immunization	Date

Section Five		**Health Insurance**	

Insurance Company	Member Number	Group/Policy Number	Customer Service
Member Hospital	Agent Name	Agent Number	Notes
Insurance Company	Member Number	Group/Policy Number	Customer Service

Member Hospital	Agent Name	Agent Number	Notes

Section Six	What I want an Emergency Physician to Know About My Child

What you need to know about my Child's Medical History

What you need to know about my Child's Personality

These are my Child's Likes and Dislikes

What Calms Her or Him Down

These are my child's Food Preferences and Bedtime Routines

Anything else I want you to know about my child

Section Seven	Recent Medical Procedures and Tests

Procedure 1	Date	Reason for Procedure
Physician	Hospital	Results
Procedure 2	Date	Reason for Procedure
Physician	Hospital	Results

Medical Test 1	Date	Reason for Procedure
Physician	Hospital	Results
Medical Test 2	Date	Reason for Procedure
Physician	Hospital	Results

Section Eight	Alternative Medicines and Other Substances Commonly Used

Vitamins or Herbs Taken	Dosage	Frequency/Last Occurrence/Notes
Vitamins or Herbs Taken	Dosage	Frequency/Last Occurrence/Notes
Vitamins or Herbs Taken	Dosage	Frequency/Last Occurrence/Notes

Section Nine	Counselors or Other Health Providers

Counselor 1	Specialty	Phone	Alternate Phone
Counselor 2	Specialty	Phone	Alternate Phone

Family Emergency Plan

Meeting Place:

Contact Name/#

Out of Town Contact:

IM/Twitter:

Alternate Meeting Place:

Notes:

THE BACKUP PLAN Grab it and Go Emergency Card

Name:

Birth Yr/Blood Type:

Physician:

Contact:

Contact:

Allergies:

See ICE info in: My Cell phone

< FOLD HERE >

Family Emergency Plan

Meeting Place:

Contact Name/#

Out of Town Contact:

IM/Twitter:

Alternate Meeting Place:

Notes:

THE BACKUP PLAN Grab it and Go Emergency Card

Name:

Birth Yr/Blood Type:

Physician:

Contact:

Contact:

Allergies:

See ICE info in: My Cell phone

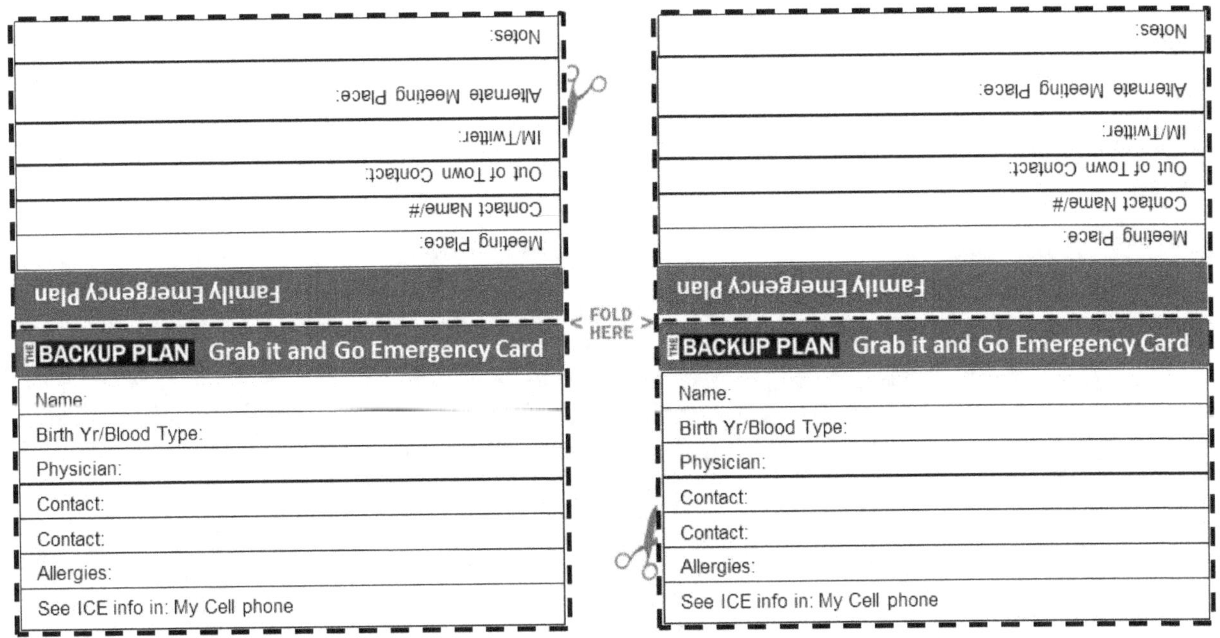

Family Emergency Plan

Meeting Place:

Contact Name/#

Out of Town Contact:

IM/Twitter:

Alternate Meeting Place:

Notes:

THE BACKUP PLAN Grab it and Go Emergency Card

Name:

Birth Yr/Blood Type:

Physician:

Contact:

Contact:

Allergies:

See ICE info in: My Cell phone

< FOLD HERE >

Family Emergency Plan

Meeting Place:

Contact Name/#

Out of Town Contact:

IM/Twitter:

Alternate Meeting Place:

Notes:

THE BACKUP PLAN Grab it and Go Emergency Card

Name:

Birth Yr/Blood Type:

Physician:

Contact:

Contact:

Allergies:

See ICE info in: My Cell phone

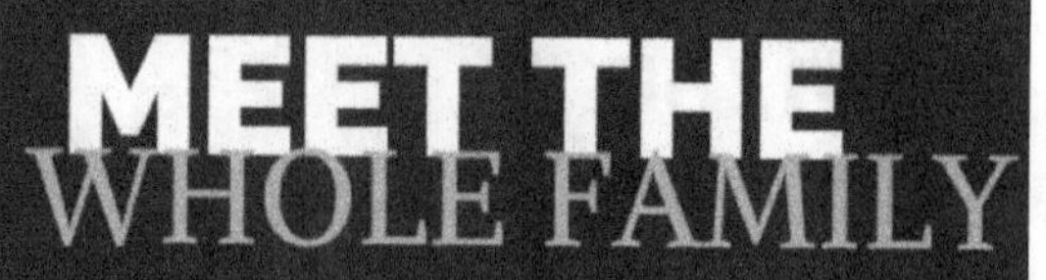

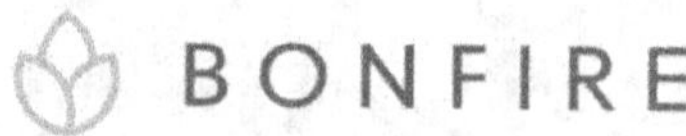

A percentage of each product sold will go towards putting our newest book *#Alone Together*, into the hands of the families who need it. The book's mission? To help keep hospitalized COVID-19 patients from dying alone, by giving their families the tools they need to stay connected with them and their medical team.

To purchase masks, mugs & tee shirts   https://www.bonfire.com/store/getyourstufftogether/
To purchase phone cases   https://www.zazzle.com/s/wealthoftulips+phone+cases

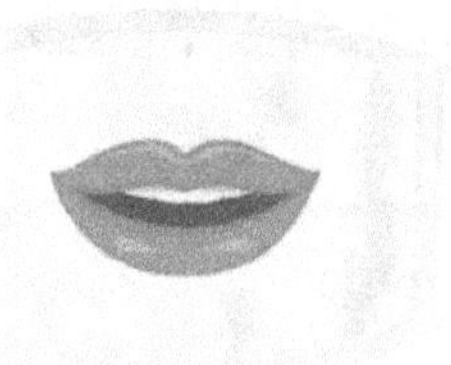

Richly Red Smile Mask

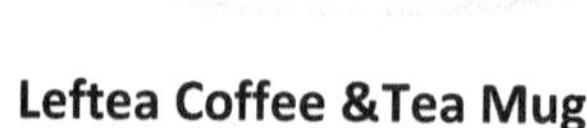

Creativi-Tea Coffee &Tea Mug

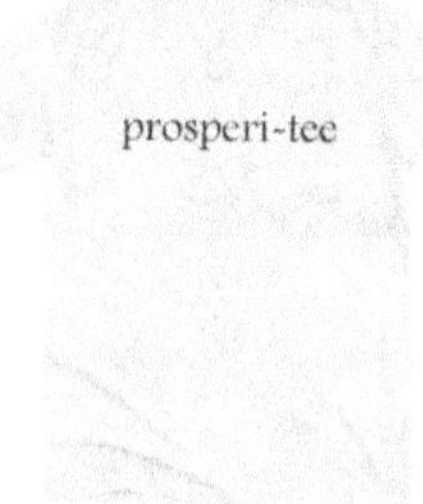

Prosperi-Tee Tee Shirt

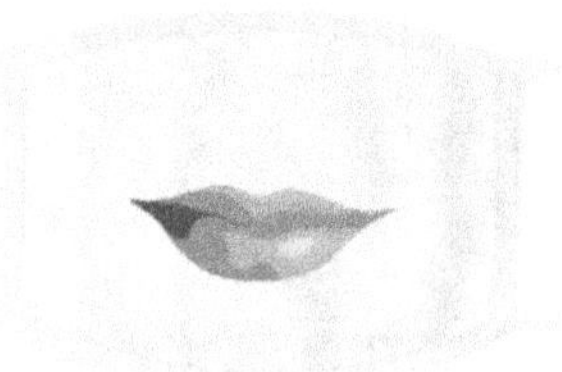

Pretty In Pink Smile Mask

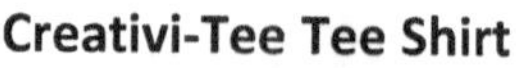

Leftea Coffee &Tea Mug

Creativi-Tee Tee Shirt

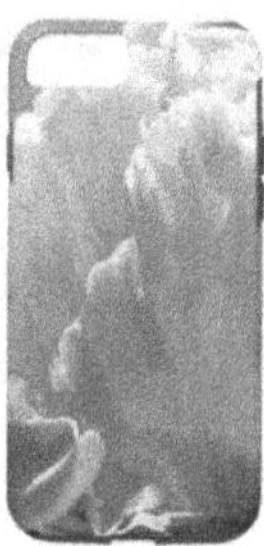

Red Parrot Tulip Phone Case

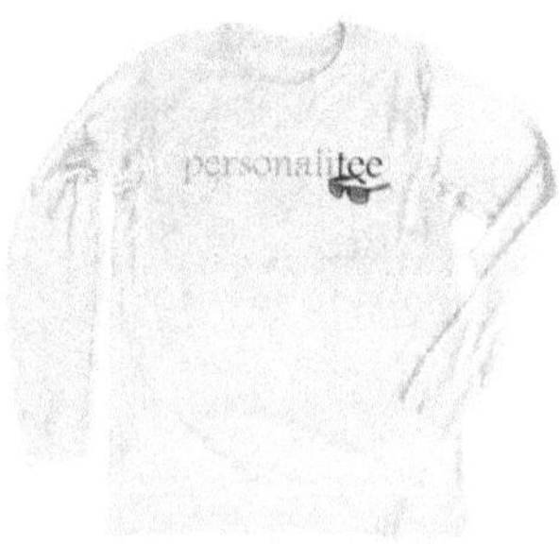

Personali-Tee Tee Shirt

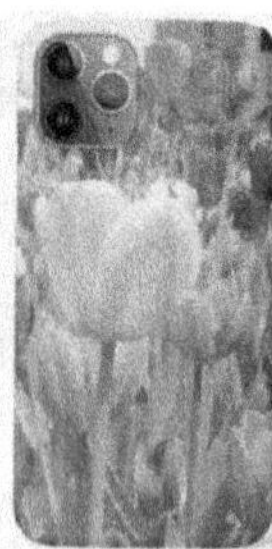

Tulips In Breeze Phone Case

About The Authors

Janet and Laura are one of the only mother/daughter writing teams in the entertainment industry. They began their careers in production on network sitcoms at MGM and Warner Bros and are currently developing their own original movies and television series.

The Greenwalds were introduced to emergency preparedness the hard way, when a jumbo-jet crashed across the street from their home. But it was a horrendous medical tragedy – one that took the life of their mother/grandmother, Elaine Sullivan – that propelled them into new territory.

When Elaine's hospital failed to notify Jan and Laura of her hospitalization they were not only prevented from being at her side, but they were also kept from preventing the drug interaction that took Elaine's life.

After uncovering a loophole in the laws which regulate the notification of the next of kin of hospital patients, Laura & Jan joined forces with legislators in Illinois and California to enact three Next of Kin Laws, before creating Notify In 7, a training program that provides hospital professionals with the skills they need to notify and reunite trauma victims with their loved ones, quickly and easily.   Hoping to keep other families from experiencing the same thing they had, they turned their story into a screenplay called Without Consent, now in development as a feature film.

Their book *Keep Everything You Love Safe*, gives readers quick and easy steps they can take to keep everything that's important to them organized, safe and accessible. Each section – over 30 in all – covers a different area from backing up & fixing family photos, home movies and music, to creating an evacuation plan, securing vital documents, medical information, financial information and data.

Between their books, blog and website, over 1.5 million people have used Jan and Laura's shortcut sheets, action plans and materials to keep themselves, their homes, their families and the things that they love, safe and secure.

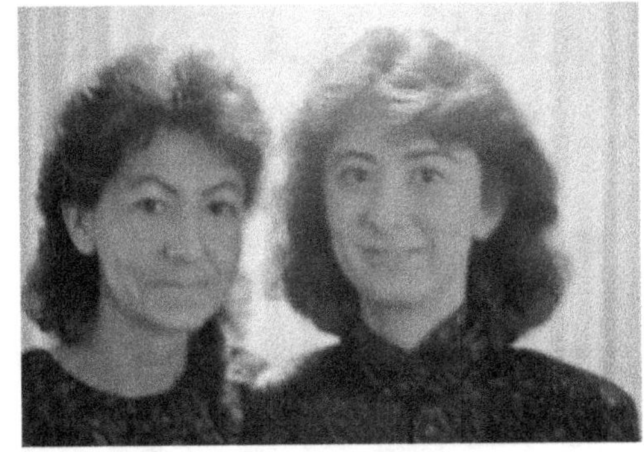